D1446605

The Definitive Guide to Back, Joint, and Nerve Pain Relief!

How the RESTORE-CARE™ Protocol Is Treating Chronic Pain Without Drugs, Shots Or Surgery And How You Can Start Living The Active, Pain-Free Life You Deserve.

Dr. Michael Santo, DPT
Dr. Stephen Lembo, DC
Dr. Brian Crane, DPT

Contents

1 What You Need to Know about Peripheral
   Neuropathy. 7

2 What You Need to Know About Back
   and Neck Pain. 16

3 What You Need to Know About Knee Pain,
   Even If You're "Bone on Bone". 40

4 Low Level Light Therapy And Class IV
   Lasers – Can It Help You? 58

5 Electrotherapy for Pain Relief and Nerve
   Re-education? 66

6 Spinal Decompression For Herniated,
   Bulging Degenerated Discs, Spinal
   Stenosis and Sciatica 73

7 Knee Decompression for Knee Pain and
   Osteoarthritis. 85

8 Soft Tissue Therapy That Keeps You Moving! . . . 93

9 Good Health Starts with Good Nutrition. 100

10 Getting Back to the Basics of Wellness 112

11 Success Stories 117

Bibliography 158

Dedication

This book is dedicated to the families of the
authors, for their unwavering love and support
personally and in all our professional careers
– we couldn't have done it without you!

And to all our patients, current and past, whose
loyalty and trust in us does not go unnoticed.

You are the reason we get up each and
every day with the energy and passion
to fulfill our one common goal:

To help our communities get their
lives back, one patient at a time!

CHAPTER 1

What You Need to Know about Peripheral Neuropathy

What is Peripheral Neuropathy? It helps to break the term down and look at each individual word. **Neuropathy** refers to pain that is caused by nerve damage. The **peripheral** part of the term refers to the peripheral nervous system – that's all of the nerves in your body that radiate out from your spinal cord. So peripheral neuropathy is typically presented as pain and tingling caused by nerve damage in the extremities.

The most common areas affected by peripheral neuropathy are the nerves in the extremities, like your arms, hands, legs, and feet. People with peripheral neuropathy generally describe the pain as stabbing, tingling, numbness, burning, or icy coldness. Many of these patients also report some weakness in the affected area.

Neuropathy of the small fiber nerves reduces sensation and can cause the patient not to be able to feel cuts, burns, punctures, or blisters on the skin. Reduced sensation in the feet can cause car accidents when people fail to sense whether they are pressing the gas pedal or the brake, or they may not be able to regulate the pressure they apply to a pedal.

Neuropathy of the large fiber nerves in the legs can cause loss of balance and coordination. This type of neuropathy causes thousands of falls every year. A fall puts the patient at risk for hip fractures, head traumas, and other serious injuries.

In addition to the extremities, other parts of the body can be affected by neuropathy; for example, the peripheral nervous system also controls your vital organs. Damage to the associated nerves can cause heartburn, indigestion, difficulty swallowing, constipation, and many other problems.

What Causes Peripheral Neuropathy?

Instead of delving into the hundreds of specific causes there are for peripheral neuropathy, we will break them down into three general categories.

1. **Circulation related peripheral neuropathy** is most often experienced by people with diabetes, but anyone with reduced blood circulation is at risk. When the small blood vessels surrounding the nerves die off, the nerves are deprived of nourishment and will also eventually die. The damaged nerves are the source of the pain and tingling.

   Over 50% of diabetics develop some form of neuropathy (Mayo Clinic). Peripheral neuropathy is also the top cause of amputations for diabetics.

2. **Toxicity related peripheral neuropathy** can be caused by any sort of exposure to toxins.

The two causes we typically focus on are chemotherapy drugs and statins.

a. **Chemotherapy-induced peripheral neuropathy** is a side effect reported by many cancer patients. Some chemotherapy drugs are more likely to cause neuropathy than others. Patients who are on a more frequent treatment schedule are also more likely to experience neuropathy.

b. **Statin-induced peripheral neuropathy** is caused by the use of drugs that doctors prescribe to reduce fats, including triglycerides and cholesterol, in the blood.

3. **Trauma induced peripheral neuropathy** is caused by events like car accidents, falls, or athletic injuries. Any of these events can cause damage to the peripheral nerves. Wearing a cast, walking with crutches, or frequent repetitive motions can also damage nerves. (Mayo Clinic)

One important fact to realize is that regardless of the cause of peripheral neuropathy, the damage is the same under a microscope. The techniques for rebuilding the nerves do not change.

How Do You Treat Peripheral Neuropathy?

Medical doctors routinely tell their patients that nerves cannot regenerate themselves, but it's simply not true! Several treatments have been proven to stimulate the growth of the nerve endings and the blood vessels that nourish them.

If the symptoms are caused by a treatable underlying condition, it is almost always possible to reverse the neuropathy. While medications can reduce the pain associated with peripheral neuropathy, painkillers do nothing to repair or reverse the damage to the nerves and blood vessels. Getting to the root cause of the neuropathy and taking steps to reverse the damage is the only effective and long-lasting method of treatment.

The end goal in treating peripheral neuropathy is to remove blockage so that the nerves can function properly and send and receive messages with the brain. The best way to achieve this is with a comprehensive treatment plan. That's why we use several methods concurrently to treat our peripheral neuropathy patients. At our clinic, peripheral neuropathy appointments last about 45 minutes rather than the standard 15-minute visit.

Our Nerve-Restore™ Treatment Protocol: A Modern Approach to Treating Neuropathy.

Low Level Light Therapy (LLLT) – LLLT uses low-power lasers or infrared light-emitting diodes to promote nerve growth, reduce pain, improve immune response, accelerate healing of wounds and .fractures, increase collagen and DNA production, and promote fibroblast activity.

ReBuilder System – Uses a patented wave form providing electrical stimulation of the muscles to improve blood flow and normalize deficits in nerve conduction velocity. The ReBuilder System is trusted by all four Cancer Treatment Centers of America locations to alleviate chemotherapy-induced peripheral neuropathy. Most of their cancer patients who use the Re-Builder System have reduced or stopped taking their pain medicine, as they report drastically reduced pain in their extremities after treatments.

Soft Tissue Therapy – Hand-held soft tissue machines are used to massage the tissue surrounding the areas affected by peripheral neuropathy. Soft tissue therapy targets injured muscles and soft tissue. Massage, pressure, stretching and trigger point techniques are used to promote the restoration of function, improved circulation, and breaking down scar tissue.

Spinal Decompression – When peripheral neuropathy has resulted from compressed discs or restricted vertebrae, spinal decompression and joint mobilization can provide relief. Spinal decompression is a treatment technology that helps take the pressure off the discs and allow the discs to move back into place. It also stimulates blood flow, which produces a healing response. If the spinal joints are restricted, gentle specific mobilization of that spinal region can help take the pressure off the affected nerves.

We also utilize physical therapy to identify and treat problematic areas along the nerve pathway. Research has shown strengthening exercises for peripheral neuropathy moderately improve muscle strength and reduce pain. Balance and stability issues can also be addressed along with improving fine motor skills.

Each intricate part of our Nerve-Restore™ treatment protocol is equally important. Each one relies on the other to do its job. There are a lot of treatments out there that only addresses one or two of the areas mentioned above. Our goal is to create lasting change for neuropathy sufferers with a more complete approach.

These treatment methods will be discussed in more detail in the following chapters.

What Else Can I Do to Reduce My Pain?

There are additional optional components of the Nerve-Restore™ treatment protocol that cannot be controlled in the clinic setting. We provide our patients with the resources to decide for themselves if they include the following home recommendation guidelines:

Nutrition – Committing to dietary changes that reduce inflammation in the body can make a tremendous difference in peripheral neuropathy symptoms. Basically, an anti-inflammatory diet promotes foods that inhibit inflammation (fruits, vegetables, lean omega-3 rich foods) and limits the intake of foods that promote inflammation (sugars, starches, omega-6 foods).

Supplements – Natural Nitric Oxide Boosters is an intricate part of treating peripheral neuropathy. In the following chapters, we will take a closer look at the peripheral neuropathy treatment technologies we offer as part of our Nerve-Restore™ treatment protocol.

What You Need to Know About Back and Neck Pain

Arthritis (Back)

Arthritis is when there is a chronic inflammation, degeneration, and irritation of the joint. Inflammatory arthritis produces large amounts of swelling to the joint and can lead to immense amounts of pain if left untreated.

Degenerative arthritis is a wearing down of the cartilage that is used to keep our joints from degenerating. Even though this does not cause a significant amount of outward swelling, pain can occur through the friction that occurs when the cartilage has worn away. As a result, there will be stiffness in the joint, which typically becomes worse overnight when the person is the least active.

Our goal in treating degenerative arthritis is to create a less painful life for the patient overall. We would like to see an increase in flexibility, mobility, and improved strength in the areas affected by arthritis. As far as inflammatory arthritis, the goal is to reduce inflammation in the area, to reduce or eliminate pain altogether.

Sciatica

Sciatica is a radiating pain along the pathway of the sciatic nerve. This pain starts at the lower back and branches out to the hips and buttocks, and down the leg. Sciatica consists of leg pain, which might feel like a bad cramp, or it can be entirely more excruciating, making standing/sitting almost unbearable. Sciatica can occur at random, or it can develop slowly, making it harder to diagnose. You might also feel weakness, numbness, burning or tingling. It is often described as a "pins and needles" sensation down the leg. Symptoms that aren't as common might include the inability to bend the knee, or move your foot. Typically, sciatica only affects one side of the body.

What Causes Sciatica?

Sciatica is caused by a pinched nerve, most often due to a herniated disc in your spine or because of a bone spur on your vertebrae.

Symptoms of Sciatica

Pain that radiates from the lower back to your buttock and down the back of your leg

- Pain in the buttocks and/or leg that worsens when sitting
- Pain can be mild to excruciating
- Burning and/or tingling down the leg
- Weakness, numbness or difficulty moving the leg or foot
- A constant pain on one side of the buttocks
- A shooting pain that makes it difficult to stand up

- Symptoms that may constitute a medical emergency include: progressive weakness in the legs and/or bladder/bowel changes including incontinence

Nerve pain is caused by a mixture of pressure and inflammation on the nerve root. Treatment is focused on relieving both of these conditions.[1]

Disc Problems

If you've ever experienced a damaged spinal disc, you understand the high level of pain it can bring. The simplest movement can make it worse or downright excruciating. Spinal discs are round, rubbery pads that go between the vertebrae and are made up of two parts: the elastic outer shell (annulus fibrosis), and the jelly-like contents (nucleus pulposus). The outer shell can handle quite a lot of pressure without damage, but certain types of injuries can damage the shell and push its contents out.

Ninety percent of disc injuries are in the lumbar region of the lower back. Though most herniated discs put pressure on surrounding nerves causing pain, it is possible to have deformed discs without pain and discomfort. Herniated discs are most common in men and women who are 30 to 50 years old, however, active children and younger adults may also experience disc problems. People who exercise regularly are much less likely to experience disc issues as they tend to stay flexible longer.

When a patient has a symptomatic disc (one that presents with low back pain and/or leg pain), it is the disc space itself that is the source of pain. These discs have a number of important functions including shock absorption, keeping the vertebral column stable and giving the vertebrae 'pivot points' to allow movement.

What Causes Disc Problems?

When a disc is stressed, its inner "jelly-like" material begins to swell and eventually start to ooze out of its tougher, outer membrane. If the disc becomes severely injured, all or part of the core material may push through the outer casing at a weak spot, putting pressure on surrounding nerves. Although any trauma to the lower back can bring on a disc problem, most are due to degeneration caused by aging, and the reduced flexibility that typically accompanies it. Poor muscle tone and posture are contributing factors to disc problems, as is obesity. In severe cases, insufficient collagen is thought to be at fault. However, sometimes a disc swells or tears on its own without any known cause.

Symptoms of Disc Problems

The symptoms of a damaged disc can vary according to its location and severity. Many people who show evidence on scanning of damaged discs have no symptoms. However, general signs may include:

- Back pain
- Pain radiating down the legs
- Worsening pain associated with bending over or sitting down for a long time

- Worsening pain associated with activities like coughing or sneezing
- Pain worsens at night
- Pain when walking short distances
- Numbness or pins-and-needles in an arm or leg.[2]

How Do You Treat Back Pain?

You are having severe back pain, so you go to your doctor to find out what's wrong. You are told it **could** be a "pinched nerve" or a pulled muscle, or arthritis and you are given medications to "see if that takes care of it, if it doesn't, come back and see me." Weeks go by and you are *still* suffering, so you go back. This time your doctor sends you to a specialist, maybe a neurosurgeon or orthopedic surgeon.

If you are lucky, the neurosurgeon tells you that you are probably not a surgical candidate (yet) and prescribes physical therapy to "see if that takes care of it." Months go by and you are still suffering, so now you go back to see him, and this time you want results! At last, he prescribes steroid injections or "epidurals" to "see if that takes care of it" and amazingly, you actually feel some relief!

For a few weeks *(or if you are lucky – months)* you feel like a new person, until one day you feel that ever-familiar twinge in your lower back. Slowly but surely the symptoms reappear. So, you go back again to the neurosurgeon to get another injection, and this time it doesn't last as long. And you go back again for another injection... so on and so on. There are some people who go back 5, 6, even **8** times! Until one day, instead of giving you another injection...

He or she now tells you there are no other options and that you may have to have surgery after all...

Our Spine-Restore™ Treatment Protocol – A Modern Approach to Treating Back Pain

High Intensity Laser Therapy (HILT) – Class IV HILT – Stimulates healing at the cellular level. This is achieved by providing energy to the cells through light waves. The wavelength of a Class IV laser can penetrate deeply into tissues of the back where the pain is stemming from. Pain reduction, inflammation reduction and speeding up recovery time – all done with this non-invasive, drug-free technology.

ReBuilder System – Uses a patented wave form providing electrical stimulation of the muscles to help decrease low back pain and normalize deficits in nerve conduction velocity.

Soft Tissue Therapy – Hand-held soft tissue machines are used to massage the tissue surrounding the low back area. Soft tissue therapy targets injured muscles and soft tissue. Massage, pressure, stretching and trigger point techniques are used to promote the restoration of function, improved circulation, and breaking down scar tissue.

Spinal Decompression – When back pain has resulted from compressed discs or restricted vertebrae, spinal decompression and joint mobilization can provide relief. Spinal decompression is a treatment technology that helps to take the pressure off the discs and allow the discs to move back into place. It also stimulates blood flow, which produces a healing response.

We also utilize physical therapy to gently stretch and strengthen the supporting structures of the back as well as improve balance, stability and function.

Each intricate part of our Spine-Restore™ treatment protocol is equally important. Each one relies on the other to do its job. There are a lot of treatments out there that only address 1 or 2 of the areas mentioned above. Our goal is to create lasting change for back pain sufferers with a more complete approach.

These treatment methods will be discussed in more detail in the following chapters.

What Else Can I Do to Reduce My Pain?

There are additional optional components of the Spine-Restore™ treatment protocol that cannot be controlled in the clinic setting. We provide our patients with the resources to decide for themselves, if they want to include the following home recommendation guidelines:

Nutrition – Committing to dietary changes that reduce inflammation in the body can make a tremendous difference in back pain symptoms. Basically, an anti-inflammatory diet promotes foods that inhibit inflammation (fruits, vegetables, lean omega-3 rich foods) and limits the intake of foods that promote inflammation (sugars, starches, omega-6 foods).

In the following chapters, we will take a closer look at the back pain treatment options that we offer as part of the Spine-Restore™ treatment protocol.

Arthritis of the Neck

Arthritis is one of the most common chronic conditions causing stiffness and pain. In fact, there are more than 100 types of arthritis.[3] Arthritis causes chronic irritation, degeneration, and inflammation of a joint or multiple joints. There are both inflammatory and degenerative forms of this condition. Inflammatory arthritis produces an uncomfortable amount of swelling of the joints. It can lead to a lot of pain and create erosive changes in the joint if left untreated.

Degenerative arthritis is a wearing down of the cartilage used to protect our joints. While this does not cause an incredible amount of swelling, there can be pain as a result of the cartilage breaking down, and the diminished joint support. The degenerative changes will cause stiffness in the joint, which is often made worse overnight because of the lack of movement to the area during the night.

What Causes Arthritis in the Neck?

Getting older can be a pain in the neck...literally! Age is the number one factor in arthritis of the neck as degeneration in the cervical vertebrae occurs in practically everyone as we age.

Symptoms of Arthritis in the Neck

- Neck pain and stiffness, especially in the morning and end of the day

- Headache that originates in the neck
- Pain in arms and shoulders
- Pain, stiffness and inability to bend the neck and fully turn the head
- Grinding noise or sensation when the neck is turned

Mechanical Neck Pain

Mechanical neck pain is a result of degenerative disc disease and arthritis of the facet joints of the cervical spine.

Mechanical neck pain is a condition that can become chronic due to degenerative disc disease and arthritis in the neck, with the source of pain coming from the spine and its structure. This happens when one of the joints in the spinal area loses its normal resiliency and shock absorption. When a joint becomes dysfunctional, its normal range of movement may be affected and it can be rather painful.

Dysfunctional joints may turn into muscle pain, and even affect the nervous system. This may happen because of the high amount of nerve receptors in the joint. Any muscles related to the joint can become tense and under-active. The muscle imbalance can cause additional stress on the joint, aggravating the joint dysfunction that exists already. Nearly any joint in the spine, from the neck all the way down to the sacroiliac joints, can cause pain. When the joints aren't being used on a regular basis, degenerative pain occurs.

What Causes Mechanical Neck Pain?

- Degenerative issues with the cervical spine, the mechanical parts that allow us to move our head up and down and around
- Minor strains or sprains to muscles or ligaments in the neck
- Bad posture. For example, neck pain is more common in people who spend much of their working day at a desk, with a 'bent-forward' posture.
- Sometimes the exact cause is unknown.

Symptoms of Mechanical Neck Pain

- Mechanical Neck Pain will not only induce pain in the neck, but also in the shoulders, and upper back
- Headaches
- Spasms
- Neck pain tends to worsen with movement

Neck Pain due to Whiplash

Whiplash syndrome is a collection of symptoms that result when there is soft-tissue injury of the cervical spine. Whiplash is very common whenever the head is forcefully jerked forward, back, or both. It is a common injury with automobile accidents. In fact, many people have suffered whiplash even in low impact car collisions. It is also common for someone to have a delayed onset of whiplash, where the person does not realize that they have had a whiplash injury. When this occurs, usually at some future point in time, that patient will begin to present with some of the classic signs of a whiplash injury.

What Causes Neck Pain from Whiplash?

The rapid and forceful movement that jerks the head forward and back causes major strain to the cervical spine. Though most often associated with a rear-end collision, whiplash can also occur from a sports injury, physical abuse or trauma.

The most common whiplash symptoms are:

- Neck pain and/or stiffness
- Blurred vision
- Difficulty swallowing
- Irritability
- Fatigue
- Dizziness
- Pain between the shoulder blades
- Pain in the arms or legs, feet and hands
- Headache
- Low back pain and/or stiffness
- Shoulder pain
- Nausea
- Ringing in the ears
- Vertigo

- Numbness and tingling
- Pain in the jaw or face

Cervical Herniated Disc

The back is composed of bones, joints, discs, ligaments and muscles. The bones that run from the neck down the spine are called vertebrae. In between each vertebra is a disc. These discs have three main functions:

1. Act as a shock absorber between adjoining vertebrae.
2. Act as joints that allow for mobility in the spine.
3. Act as ligaments that hold the vertebrae of the spine together.

In order for a disc to function properly, it must have high water content because this makes the disc strong yet flexible. As long as the disc is well hydrated and undamaged, it has the ability to support heavy loads.

Injury, poor body mechanics and poor nutrition can cause the disc to become dehydrated. This causes the disc to lose its ability to support the spinal bones during everyday living. This can result in disc injury such as a bulge or herniation.

When a cervical (neck) disc becomes herniated, it can cause pain in the neck, shoulders, chest, arms or hands. Arm pain from a cervical herniated disc is one of the more common cervical spine conditions found in the 30 to 50-year-old age group. Even though a herniated disc may happen due to some form of injury or trauma to the cervical spine, more often than not, the symptoms seem to appear rather spontaneously. Arm pain due to a cervical herniated disc occurs because the disc material presses or pinches on a cervical nerve, causing pain to radiate down the nerve pathway of the entire arm. In addition to pain, a person may experience weakness, numbness, and tingling in the arm.

The two most common levels in the cervical spine to herniate are the C5 – C6 level (cervical 5 and cervical 6) and the C6 – C7 level. (Take a look at the figure on the next page for a reference point)

The next most common is the C4 – C5 level. The least likely cervical herniation would occur at the C7 – T1 level. The nerve that winds up being affected by the disc herniation is the one exiting the spine at that level, so at the C5 – C6 level, it is the C6 nerve root that is affected. (Take a look at the figure on the next page for a reference point.)

Human vertebral column

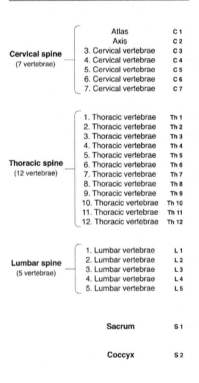
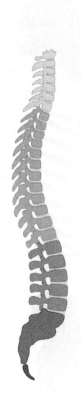

Cervical spine (7 vertebrae)	Atlas	C 1
	Axis	C 2
	3. Cervical vertebrae	C 3
	4. Cervical vertebrae	C 4
	5. Cervical vertebrae	C 5
	6. Cervical vertebrae	C 6
	7. Cervical vertebrae	C 7
Thoracic spine (12 vertebrae)	1. Thoracic vertebrae	Th 1
	2. Thoracic vertebrae	Th 2
	3. Thoracic vertebrae	Th 3
	4. Thoracic vertebrae	Th 4
	5. Thoracic vertebrae	Th 5
	6. Thoracic vertebrae	Th 6
	7. Thoracic vertebrae	Th 7
	8. Thoracic vertebrae	Th 8
	9. Thoracic vertebrae	Th 9
	10. Thoracic vertebrae	Th 10
	11. Thoracic vertebrae	Th 11
	12. Thoracic vertebrae	Th 12
Lumbar spine (5 vertebrae)	1. Lumbar vertebrae	L 1
	2. Lumbar vertebrae	L 2
	3. Lumbar vertebrae	L 3
	4. Lumbar vertebrae	L 4
	5. Lumbar vertebrae	L 5
	Sacrum	S 1
	Coccyx	S 2

What Causes a Cervical Herniated Disc?

As we age, ligaments surrounding the discs become less flexible and elastic, making them brittle and more easily torn. This can also prevent important nutrients and hydration to get to the disc to keep it healthy. When a disc herniates, it puts pressure on nearby spinal nerves or the spinal cord, and this is what causes all that pain.

Symptoms of a Cervical Herniated Disc

- Neck, shoulder and/or arm pain
- pain ranges from dull, aching and hard to locate to sharp, burning and easy to pinpoint
- radiating arm pain
- numbness, tingling, or weakness in the arm or hand in more severe cases

A specific cervical disc herniation has its own pain patterns and neurological problems. These are as follows:

- **C5 (C5 nerve root):** Can cause weakness in the deltoid muscle in the upper arm. Does not usually cause numbness or tingling. Can cause shoulder pain.

- **C6 (C6 nerve root):** Can cause weakness in the biceps (muscles in the front of the upper arms) and wrist extensor muscles. Numbness and tingling along with pain can radiate to the thumb side of the hand. This is one of the most common levels for a cervical disc herniation to occur.

- **C7 (C7 nerve root):** Can cause weakness in the triceps (muscles in the back of the upper arm and extending to the forearm) and the finger extensor muscles. Numbness and tingling along with pain can radiate down the triceps and into the middle finger. This is also one of the most common levels for a cervical disc herniation.

- **T1 (C8 nerve root):** Can cause weakness with handgrip. Numbness and tingling and pain can radiate down the arm to the pinky finger side of hand.

Our Spine-Restore™ Treatment Protocol – A Modern Approach to Treating Neck Pain

High Intensity Laser Therapy (HILT) – Class IV

HILT – Stimulates healing at the cellular level. This is achieved by providing energy to the cells through light waves. The wavelength of a Class IV laser can penetrate deeply into tissues of the neck where the pain is stemming from. Pain reduction, inflammation reduction and speeding up recovery time – all done with this non-invasive, drug-free technology.

ReBuilder System – Uses a patented wave form providing electrical stimulation of the muscles to help decrease neck pain and normalize deficits in nerve conduction velocity.

Soft Tissue Therapy – Hand-held soft tissue machines are used to massage the tissue surrounding the neck area. Soft tissue therapy targets injured muscles and soft tissue. Massage, pressure, stretching and trigger point techniques are used to promote the restoration of function, improved circulation, and breaking down scar tissue.

Spinal Decompression – When neck pain has resulted from compressed discs or restricted vertebrae, spinal decompression and joint mobilization can provide relief. Spinal decompression is a treatment technology that helps to take the pressure off the discs and allow the discs to move back into place. It also stimulates blood flow, which produces a healing response.

We also utilize physical therapy to gently stretch and strengthen the supporting structures of the neck as well as improve balance, stability and function.

Each intricate part of our Spine-Restore™ treatment protocol is equally important. Each one relies on the other to do its job. There are a lot of treatments out there that only address 1 or 2 of the areas mentioned above. Our goal is to create lasting change for neck pain sufferers with a more complete approach.

These treatment methods will be discussed in more detail in the following chapters.

What Else Can I Do to Reduce My Pain?

There are additional optional components of the Spine-Restore™ treatment protocol that cannot be controlled in the clinic setting. We provide our patients with the resources to decide for themselves, if they want to include the following home recommendation guidelines:

Nutrition – Committing to dietary changes that reduce inflammation in the body can make a tremendous difference in neck pain symptoms. Basically, an anti-inflammatory diet promotes foods that inhibit inflammation (fruits, vegetables, lean omega-3 rich foods) and limits the intake of foods that promote inflammation (sugars, starches, omega-6 foods).

In the following chapters, we will take a closer look at the neck pain treatment options that we offer as part of the Spine-Restore™ treatment protocol.

What You Need to Know About Knee Pain, Even If You're "Bone on Bone"

Knee Bursitis

A bursa is a fluid-filled sac that reduces friction, rubbing and irritation by acting as a cushion between your bones, the skin, the tendons and muscles near your joints. When the bursa becomes inflamed, this is then called bursitis. Knee bursitis is the inflammation near your knee joint. Each knee has 11 bursae but knee bursitis occurs mostly at the kneecap or inside the knee.

What Causes Knee Bursitis?

Bursitis is commonly caused by repetitive movement, overuse, minor injury or serious injury. Sustained pressure due to kneeling, such as people or workers that spend a lot of time on their knees, may be at risk. A bursa can become inflamed as the result of another condition like osteoarthritis, rheumatoid arthritis, or gout in your knee. Very rarely, about 20% of people with knee bursitis have an infected bursa. If the immune system is intensely weak, the bursa may get infected with bacteria. An infection can occur from an open cut or even a bug bite, but some are just unknown.

Symptoms of Knee Bursitis

- Tenderness and pain when pressure is put on the knee, when straightened or bent
- Inflammation
- Warmth/redness
- Swelling of the bursa
- Pressure

- Fever may be a sign of Septic bursitis (Infected bursa)[4], [5], [6]

Knee (Patellar) Tendonitis/Tendonosis

Knee (patellar) tendonitis/tendonosis is inflammation or degeneration of the patellar tendon. Tendons are structures that connect the muscle to bone. The job of the tendons is to provide the connection between muscles and bones, and allow muscles to exert force on the body part.

Patellar tendonitis is an injury to the tendon connecting your kneecap (patella) to your shinbone. The patellar tendon works with the muscles at the front of your thigh to extend your knee, making it possible to run, kick or jump. Patellar tendonosis is cartilage degeneration or chronically overused tendon with microtrauma. The tendon can tear in half, causing the tendon to rupture, making it impossible to straighten or bend the knee. Patellar tendonitis or tendonosis is also known as "jumper's knee."

What Causes Knee (Patellar) Tendonitis/Tendonosis?

Patellar tendonitis/tendonosis is caused mostly from overuse, and repetitive stress put on the patellar tendon. The repeated stress can result in the tendon tearing. As tears begin to spread, they cause pain and weakness in the knee. Activities such as running, biking, squatting, kneeling, going up or down stairs, jumping, and even walking may contribute to Knee Tendonitis/Tendonosis. The tendon may also start swelling when your knee is bent for long periods of time such as sitting in a car.

Symptoms of Knee (Patellar) Tendonitis/Tendonosis

Symptoms start off as mild and may only be present as physical activity begins. The pain will start to worsen as the physical activity becomes more demanding. Eventually, pain will become so uncomfortable that it will interfere with typical daily activities, such as standing up, climbing, walking, or even when at rest. Other symptoms include:

- Aching
- Swelling
- Grinding feeling in the kneecap
- Irritation/Inflammation
- Stiffness in the morning due to fluid leaving the tendon during rest

Tendonosis symptoms may last up to 6 months.[7],[8],[9]

Knee Meniscal Injuries

The meniscus is a rubbery C-shaped disc that acts like a cushion to the shinbone to the thighbone. Each knee has two menisci; one at the outer edge of the knee and one at the inner edge. The menisci keep the knee steady by balancing the weight across the knee. A torn meniscus can prevent the knee from working appropriately. When older people experience a meniscus tear, it's likely to be degeneration. When the cartilage in the knee becomes weak and thin due to age, it is much easier to tear. Meniscus tears are among the most common knee injuries.[10]

What are the Causes of Knee Meniscal Injuries?

Athletes who play contact sports are at risk for meniscus tears. However, you don't have to be an athlete to get a meniscus tear. The meniscus can be torn from activities with direct contact. Pressure from a twist, forced rotation, lifting heavy items, or getting up too quickly from a squatting position may all lead to a meniscus tear. Sports that contribute to having this injury are football, basketball, soccer or tennis.[11]

Symptoms of Knee Meniscal Injury

- Pain
- Swelling or stiffness
- Popping sound/sensation in the knee
- Difficulty in moving the knee
- Knee locking
- Knee giving way/unable to support the body
- Difficulty bending or straightening the knee fully[12, 13]

Chondromalacia Patellae

Chondromalacia, also known as "runner's knee," is the softening of the cartilage under the kneecap. This is due to poor alignment of the kneecap as it may slide over to the end of the thighbone. Chondromalacia patellae may develop when the knee is overused or injured.

What causes Chondromalacia?

The kneecap is usually right over the joint of the knee. When the knee bends, the movement results in the back of the kneecap gliding over the bone of the knee gracefully. However, in some people, the kneecap tends to rub against one side of the knee joint, irritating the cartilage and causing knee pain. Other causes due to improper movement of the knee joint are:

- Poor alignment
- Weak hamstrings and quadriceps
- Continuous stress to the knee joints
- A direct injury to the kneecap

Symptoms of Chondromalacia

- Sensations of grinding or cracking when bending or extending the knee
- Prolonged sitting
- Tightness or fullness in the knee area
- Front of knee pain
- Swelling and tenderness around the kneecap[14], [15]

Knee Ligament Sprains

A medial ligament sprain injury is a tear of the ligament on the inside of the knee. A knee ligament sprain happens when one or more ligaments in your knee are unexpectedly stretched or torn. Ligaments are tissues that hold bones together and support the knee to keep the joint and bones in the right position. The knee joint helps stabilize and support the knee when it is moved in different positions. There are four ligaments that help support the knee, and are prone to injury:

- **Anterior Cruciate Ligament (ACL)** – One of two major ligaments in the knee connecting to the thigh bone to the shin to the knee.

- **Posterior Cruciate Ligament (PCL)** – Second major ligament connecting to the thigh bone to the shin to the knee.

- **Lateral Collateral Ligament (LCL)** – Connects the thigh bone to the fibula (the outer/smaller of the two bones between the knee and the ankle), which is on the lower leg outside of the knee.

- **Medial Collateral Ligament (MCL)** – Connects to the thighbone to the shin bone in the side of the knee.

What are the Causes of Knee Ligament Sprains?

Knee ligament sprains are common in exercise or sports such as soccer, football, basketball, skiing, and gymnastics. Sprains can happen from a fall, or from landing with improper/twisted form. Getting directly hit on the knee, extending, jumping then landing, stopping quickly after running, not warming up before workout, or excessive exercise, can all cause knee sprains.

Symptoms of Knee Ligament Sprains

- Popping or snapping sound
- Swelling
- Pain
- Tenderness
- A feeling that your knee is unstable or giving out
- Bruising around the knee
- Stiffness or decreased movement[16], [17]

Arthritis/Arthrosis (Knee)

Arthritis is chronic inflammation, and irritation of a joint. Arthrosis is the term for a degenerative disease of the joint, caused by wear and tear on the cartilage lining the joint. Cartilage is the tissue that covers the ends of bones and helps joints move smoothly. The major types of arthritis that affect the knee are osteoarthritis and rheumatoid arthritis.

Osteoarthritis

Arthrosis is seen as a cause in the early stages of Osteoarthritis. Osteoarthritis is the most common form of arthritis, occurring when the cartilage on the ends of the bones begins to wear and tears. Osteoarthritis causes the bones of the joints to rub more closely against each other. The rubbing of the cartilage results in pain, swelling, stiffness, and bone spurs. Osteoarthritis develops slowly, gradually becoming more painful over time.

Rheumatoid Arthritis

Rheumatoid arthritis is a chronic, inflammatory disease that affects multiple joints throughout the body. Rheumatoid arthritis is an autoimmune disease, meaning that the immune system attacks its own tissues, the membrane, cartilage on the ends of your bones, and possibly even the bone.

What Causes Arthritis/ Arthrosis in the Knee?

Arthritis/Arthrosis in the knee may be caused from injury, infection, age, being overweight, or can even be hereditary.

Symptoms of Arthritis/ Arthrosis in the Knee

- Joint: reduced range of motion, pain, stiffness, tenderness, inflexibility, and swelling.
- Bones rubbing together
- Bone spurs (outgrowth of bone)
- Redness or warmth of skin around affected joints
- Decreased mobility: Having trouble walking or climbing, getting in and out of chairs/ beds.[18], [19], [20]

Iliotibial Band Friction Syndrome

The iliotibial band is the ligament that runs down the outside of the thigh from the hip to the shin. The Iliotibial band (IT band) attaches to the knee and helps stabilize and create movement in the joint. The IT band connects the pelvis, upper leg and lower back, and helps the lateral part of the knee stay stable as the joint flexes and extends. Iliotibial Band Friction Syndrome is an overuse injury. The inflammation causes pain that runs from the side of the hip to the outside of the knee, and is known to be very painful and hard to deal with. IT band syndrome is most common with athletes, especially runners.

What are the Causes of Iliotibial Band Friction Syndrome?

Causes of IT band syndrome are overuse, triggering pain on the outside of the knee. Iliotibial band syndrome is most common with long distance runners, bicyclists and other athletes where squatting is required. This is a common injury in runners that run a lot of hills. Other causes are inflexibility, bad shoes, running too many miles, incorrect running form, or improperly warming up before exercise.

Symptoms of Iliotibial Band Friction Syndrome

- Pain or swelling on the outside of the knee
- Sensation or prickling feeling from the side of the hip to the side of the knee
- Snapping or popping at the knee
- Thickening or inflammation of the band[21], [22], [23]

How Do You Treat Knee Pain?

You are having severe knee pain, so you go to your doctor to find out what's wrong. You are told it **could** be a "ligament problem" or arthritis and you are given medications to "see if that takes care of it, if it doesn't, come back and see me." Weeks go by and you are *still* suffering, so you go back. This time your doctor sends you to a specialist, maybe an orthopedic surgeon.

If you are lucky, the orthopedic surgeon tells you that you are probably not a surgical candidate (yet) and prescribes physical therapy to "see if that takes care of it." Months go by and you are still suffering, so now you go back to see him, and this time you want results! At last, he prescribes steroid injections or "gel shots" to "see if that takes care of it" and amazingly, you actually feel some relief!

For a few weeks (*or if you are lucky – months*) you feel like a new person, until one day you feel that ever-familiar twinge in your knee. Slowly but surely the symptoms reappear. So, you go back again to the ortho to get another series of injections, and this time it doesn't last as long. And you go back again for another injection... and so on and so on. There are some people who go back 5, 6, even **8** times! Until one day, instead of giving you another injection...

He or she now tells you there are no other options and that you may have to have surgery after all...

Our Knee-Restore™ Treatment Protocol – A Modern Approach to Treating Knee Pain

High Intensity Laser Therapy (HILT) – Class IV HILT – stimulates healing at the cellular level.

This is achieved by providing energy to the cells through light waves. The wavelength of a Class IV laser can penetrate deeply into tissues of the knee where the pain is stemming from. Pain reduction, inflammation reduction and speeding up recovery time – all done with this non-invasive, drug-free technology.

ReBuilder System – Uses a patented wave form providing electrical stimulation of the muscles to help decrease knee pain and normalize deficits in nerve conduction velocity.

Soft Tissue Therapy – Hand-held soft tissue machines are used to massage the tissue surrounding the knee region. Soft tissue therapy targets injured muscles and soft tissue. Massage, pressure, stretching and trigger point techniques are used to promote the restoration of function, improved circulation, and breaking down scar tissue.

Knee Decompression – When knee pain has resulted from pressure and loss of joint spaces, knee decompression and joint mobilization can provide relief. Knee decompression is a treatment technology that helps to take the pressure off the knee joint by opening the joint spaces. It also stimulates the production of healthy synovial fluid, which helps lubricate the joint and decrease pain.

We also utilize physical therapy to gently stretch and strengthen the supporting structures of the knee as well as improve the overall function of the lower extremities.

Each intricate part of our Knee-Restore™ treatment protocol is equally important. Each one relies on the other to do its job. There are a lot of treatments out there that only address 1 or 2 of the areas mentioned above. Our goal is to create lasting change for knee pain sufferers with a more complete approach.

These treatment methods will be discussed in more detail in the following chapters.

What Else Can I Do to Reduce My Pain?

There are additional optional components of the Knee-Restore™ treatment protocol that cannot be controlled in the clinic setting. We provide our patients with the resources to decide for themselves, if they want to include the following home recommendation guidelines:

Nutrition – Committing to dietary changes that reduce inflammation in the body can make a tremendous difference in knee pain symptoms. Basically, an anti-inflammatory diet promotes foods that inhibit inflammation (fruits, vegetables, lean omega-3 rich foods) and limits the intake of foods that promote inflammation (sugars, starches, omega-6 foods).

In the following chapters, we will take a closer look at the knee pain treatment options that we offer as part of the Knee-Restore™ treatment protocol.

Low Level Light Therapy And Class IV Lasers – Can It Help You?

Since lasers were invented in the 1960s, medical professionals have discovered numerous applications for lasers to improve people's health. As the technology advanced through the years, ophthalmologists, dermatologists, and surgeons quickly found lasers to be useful in treating their patients. Low level light therapy (LLLT) is in its fourth decade of use as a method of treating sprains, back and neck pain, arthritis, ulcers, and more.

Looking to the future, studies are currently being conducted to test out LLLT's effectiveness in treating sperm mobility, spinal cord injuries, stroke victims, Parkinson's patients, and Alzheimer's disease.

How Do LLLT and Class IV Lasers Work?

Think back to your high school biology class. You may recall that plants use a process called photosynthesis to produce energy. The plant changes that energy into ATP, which is the fuel stored and used by all cells in all living things – plants and animals alike. LLLT stimulates the production of enzyme cytochrome c oxidase, which, like sunlight for plants, produces ATP. With more fuel being produced, cells have more energy to repair themselves. Currently, numerous studies being conducted around the world are proving that LLLT can help the body regenerate its own tissues, including spinal cord and nerve tissues. The therapy also holds promise for restoring eyesight, reversing numerous neurological diseases, and stroke recovery.

What Else Could LLLT Treat in the Future?

Fibromyalgia is a condition that causes the brain to process pain abnormally, resulting in chronic, widespread pain and chronic fatigue. This condition affects millions of Americans and has been poorly understood and under-diagnosed, resulting in billions of dollars in cost to our health care system.

Fibromyalgia is primarily treated with medications; side effects often make the patient's symptoms even worse. But studies have already shown that LLLT helps to treat the pain and swelling of fibromyalgia.

Parkinson's Disease belongs to a group of conditions called motor system disorders, which are the result of the loss of dopamine-producing brain cells. The four primary symptoms of Parkinson's disease are tremors in the arms, legs, jaw, and face; stiffness of the limbs and trunk; slowness of movement; and impaired balance and coordination.

Many scientists think that one of the malfunctioning systems in Parkinson's disease is located in the mitochondria. These are the cellular systems/organelles that produce ATP, the energy for all the other systems of the body. They also help to detoxify the brain and body by regulating the free radicals circulating in the system.

A study by the UVA Morris K. Udall Parkinson's Research Center of Excellence showed that a single, brief treatment of LLLT increased the movement of the mitochondria in neuron cells to be similar to the level of movement in disease-free, age-matched control groups.[24]

Muscle regeneration is another area where LLLT holds great promise. LLLT has been shown to increase cellular function and regeneration, including cells that create muscle tissue. Studies are being conducted to determine if heart muscles can be regenerated using LLLT.

Medical doctors are taught that heart muscle does not regenerate. Therefore, when someone has a heart attack, doctors tell patients that the muscle that died in the attack is gone for good. However, new research shows that heart muscle can and does regenerate itself. This finding opens up new possibilities of regenerating heart muscle after a heart attack with LLLT, thereby preventing a host of complications including heart failure.

Diabetic ulcers are one of the many health risks associated with uncontrolled diabetes. Diabetic ulcers are extremely hard to cure. Due to artery abnormalities, diabetic neuropathy, and delayed wound healing, infection or gangrene of the extremities is relatively common.

Wound healing is usually taken care of efficiently by a healthy body. But diabetes is a disorder that impedes normal steps of the wound healing process. Common treatments – skin grafts, moist wound therapy, and negative pressure wound therapy – almost never work completely.

LLLT is a new treatment option for diabetic ulcers that is showing great promise. Unlike other therapies, LLLT has no side effects. In one case study, a man with a diabetic ulcer was treated for a total of 16 sessions of low-intensity laser therapy over a four-week period. During this time, the ulcer healed completely. During a follow-up period of nine months, there was no recurrence of the ulcer.[25]

What Role Does LLLT Play in Treating Peripheral Neuropathy?

Because LLLT stimulates cellular regeneration, it plays a vital role in a complete treatment plan for peripheral neuropathy patients. LLLT helps damaged nerves and their surrounding blood vessels regrow, gradually improving sensation and function for the patient. There are currently no drugs on the market that can help the body heal itself in such a way. Plus, unlike virtually all medications, there are absolutely no side effects associated with LLLT. The area may feel warm or tingly during the treatment, but there are no other reported physical sensations from LLLT patients.

When a patient visits our office for treatment of peripheral neuropathy, we apply LLLT around the hands, feet, or both and let the machine deliver the treatment for a specified amount of time.

What role does Class IV Lasers play in treating back and knee pain?

For knee and spine conditions, as part of our Knee-Restore™ protocol and Spine-Restore™ protocol respectively, we typically use Class IV Laser therapy applied to the area of pain.

Our clinical team will set the laser for appropriate wattage for your specific condition. The laser will be placed above the skin and focused on the area that requires treatment. Laser therapy is applied with constant and/or pulse setting.

No preparation is necessary when having treatment. As the patient, you may feel some heat or warmth during the laser treatment but it will not be uncomfortable. In fact, our patients often report feeling a pleasant, soothing effect. The patient will wear protective goggles for safety purposes.

Treatment time can vary depending on the size of the area being treated. Treatment time generally ranges between 5-8 minutes depending on the size of the area(s) being treated.

CHAPTER 5

Electrotherapy for Pain Relief and Nerve Re-education?

Electrotherapy is a pain management technique where small electrical currents stimulate nerves and muscles to release pain-killing chemicals such as endorphins, and prevents pain signals from being transmitted to the brain. Electrotherapy also improves nerve function by gently opening up the nerve pathways. It does not hurt your muscles or nerves, and it does not burn your skin. In our office, we rely on the ReBuilder System for patients seeking treatment for peripheral neuropathy, back, neck and knee pain. This technology is much different than a TENS unit. TENS units can actually make neuropathy worse over time.

ReBuilder is an FDA-cleared device that was designed originally to treat the pain, burning, numbness, and tingling associated with peripheral neuropathy. In fact, all of the Cancer Treatment Centers of America use ReBuilder to alleviate their patients' chemotherapy-induced neuropathy. We also use ReBuilder technology to help with certain types of back, neck and knee pain.

What Are the Benefits of ReBuilder Treatment?

ReBuilder treatments may significantly reduce the amount of pain medications needed to deal with an acute pain syndrome. It has also been used to effectively treat functional problems such as drop foot. The effects of this treatment method are cumulative, meaning that the longer you continue to use it, the better the results you will see.

ReBuilder also increases blood flow, strengthens muscles, and improves the transmission of signals within the nervous system. And when patients experience less pain at night, they tend to get a better night's sleep. This allows them to function better during the daytime and promotes cellular repair and regeneration during their restful hours.

How Do We Use ReBuilder?

We supply our patients with special conductive garments (socks/gloves) in order to deliver this patented electrical current. For some patients, improvement in pain, numbness and tingling can occur within just a few weeks of electrotherapy treatments.

How Does it Work?

All we have to do is put on the pads, turn on the system, and sit back so that the device can do its job. ReBuilder is an "intelligent" system, in that it analyzes the nerves 7.83 times per second, determines the correct amount of electrical signal, and then delivers it to the target area.[26]

The electrical current opens up the nerve pathways and promotes good signal conduction. During treatment, you may feel your muscles contract and relax – this is normal. As you progress through more and more treatments, your condition will improve and the need for electrotherapy is reduced. Throughout the treatment period, the ReBuilder will alter the amount of signal it delivers based on the condition of your nerves.

Whether your peripheral neuropathy is a side effect of statin drugs, chemotherapy treatment, diabetes, or another source, ReBuilder can help restore function and sensation to your peripheral nervous system. It's also working great for many types of back, neck and knee pain.

Why Is ReBuilder the Electrotherapy System of Choice?

Since ReBuilder hit the market, it has helped millions of patients repair their pain points from the inside out with no drugs, no surgery, and virtually no side effects. When you have dealt with problems like shortness of breath, memory loss, constipation, sleeplessness, and dizziness while on pain medications, the idea of treating the root cause of the pain and eliminating drugs from your daily routine often seems like nothing more than a fantasy. But it's totally possible – perhaps within weeks – with electrotherapy.

But the real reason we use ReBuilder for our back pain, knee pain and peripheral neuropathy patients is simple: we have seen the results first-hand. Almost all of our patients who use ReBuilder report feeling less numbness, pain, and tingling in the treated area. With blood flow and nerve function restored, patients become more mobile and stop relying on painkillers to get through the day.

Is ReBuilder Right for Me?

In our clinic, we are all about helping our patients heal from the inside out, without medications or surgery. Restore-Care™, our treatment protocol uses several modalities at once to treat our patients who are suffering from back pain, nerve pain and peripheral neuropathy because we believe in a broad-spectrum approach to treating chronic pain.

Our patients come to us in the midst of a very difficult period in their lives. They may be going through severe "bone on bone" osteoarthritis knee pain, a bulging or herniated disc in the neck or back or peripheral neuropathy. While the causes of their pain are different, we use similar methods to treat them all. Electrotherapy is one important treatment method that they all have in common.

Thousands of doctors in all types of practices prescribe the ReBuilder System for their patients. All four Cancer Treatment Centers of America offer it to their patients who are undergoing chemotherapy. And as a matter of fact, using ReBuilder *before* starting treatment can be an effective preventative measure against developing peripheral neuropathy in the first place.[27]

If you are suffering from the effects of back pain, knee pain or peripheral neuropathy, there is an excellent chance that ReBuilder can help. The ReBuilder is only one piece of the puzzle in our innovative Restore-Care™ program. We strongly believe that a more complete approach to chronic pain is a smarter plan of action. That's why we prescribe electrotherapy, low level light therapy or Class IV laser, rehab, and in some cases, spinal decompression therapy and nutrition to our patients who are struggling to get their pain under control and live an active life like they desire.

CHAPTER 6

Spinal Decompression For Herniated, Bulging Degenerated Discs, Spinal Stenosis and Sciatica

Back pain affects 8 out of 10 people at some point in time.[28]

Here are a few facts about low back pain:

- 80 percent of Americans experience back pain at some point during their lives.
- 46 percent of Americans surveyed by Consumer Reports indicated that lower-back pain interfered with their sleep.
- More than half the people who suffer from back pain say the pain has severely limited

their everyday activities for a week or longer at some point in time.[29]

Stat Fact: Low back pain is estimated to result in 175.8 million days of restricted activity per year.[30]

Low back pain can even be the cause of permanent disability. The cost of back pain in the U.S. is conservatively estimated to be upwards of $90 billion, according to the latest research study published in the journal *Spine*.[31]

What Causes Back Pain?

The back is composed of bones, joints, discs, ligaments and muscles. Therefore, back pain can come from problems with any of these structures. For instance, you can sprain ligaments, strain muscles, rupture discs and irritate joints. Most people think of injuries or accidents as the cause of back pain, but even simple movements such as picking something up off the floor can have painful results.

Another cause of low back pain is aging. Everyone knows about the aging process – graying hair, wrinkles and achy bones. What typically is not thought of is how our spine ages. Through the years, everyday wear and tear, as well as problems due to injuries and accidents, our spine begins to break down and degenerate. In fact, at least 30% of people between the ages of 30-50 years old will have some degree of disc degeneration.[32]

Anatomy of the Low Back

Important structures of the low back that can be related to symptoms there include the vertebrae, discs between the vertebrae, ligaments around the spine and discs, spinal cord and nerves, and muscles of the low back.

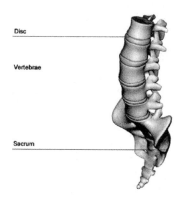

Words Defined: Lumbar Spine

The lower section of the spine, also called the low back, comprised of five large vertebrae supporting the upper body, torso and low back.

The low back or lumbar spine is made up of five bones or vertebrae with discs between each vertebra. The vertebrae are "stacked" together and provide a moveable structure that provides support while also protecting the spinal cord. The lumbar vertebrae stack immediately atop the sacrum bone that is situated in between the buttocks. On each side, the sacrum meets the iliac bone of the pelvis to form the sacroiliac joint of the buttocks.

Ligaments are strong fibrous soft tissues that firmly attach bones to bones. Ligaments attach each of the vertebrae to each other and surround each of the discs.

The nerves that provide sensation and stimulate the muscles of the low back, as well as the thighs, legs, feet and toes, exit the lumbar spinal column through bony portals, each of which is called a "foramen."

Many muscle groups that are responsible for flexing, extending and rotating the waist, as well as moving the lower extremities, attach to the lumbar spine through tendon insertions.

The discs are pads that serve as "cushions" between the individual vertebral bodies. They help to minimize the impact of stress forces on the spinal column. Each disc is designed like a jelly donut with a central softer component (nucleus pulposus) and a surrounding outer ring (annulus fibrosus). The central portion of the disc is capable of rupturing (herniating) through the outer ring, causing pain.

Functions of the Vertebral Disc

The disc has three main functions:

1. Act as a shock absorber between adjoining vertebrae
2. Act as joints that allow for mobility in the spine
3. Act as ligaments that hold the vertebrae of the spine together

In order for a disc to function properly, it must have high water content because this makes the disc strong yet flexible. As long as the disc is well hydrated and undamaged, it has the ability to support heavy loads.

Injury, poor body mechanics and poor nutrition can cause the disc to become dehydrated. This causes the disc to lose its ability to support the spinal bones during everyday living. This can result in disc injury such as a bulge or herniation.

The Cause of Disc Pain

The discs, located between vertebrae, are made up of two parts: the outer ring-like structure made up of cartilage that contains nerves (annulus fibrosus) and the gel-like interior (nucleus pulposus).

Low back pain can be caused by either bulging or herniated discs. A bulging disc means 50% or more of a disc is being squeezed to beyond its boundaries, much like a large burger extending outside of the bun. This places pressure on the highly sensitive nerve roots resulting in pain.

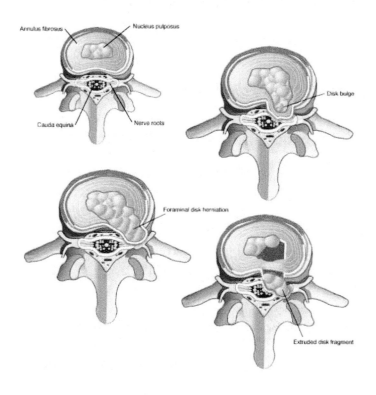

A herniation is when the gel-like substance of the nucleus oozes out of the disc, pressing against a nerve after the outer structure ruptures. Herniated discs are also known as ruptured discs, blown discs or slipped discs. The leakage of material can cause irritation to the nerve root causing LBP and even leg pain.

What is Spinal Decompression?

Spinal decompression therapy uses a medical technology that applies a distraction force to the targeted compressed disc. This gently pulls the spine apart, elongating it and creating a small vacuum between the vertebrae, which pulls the disc back into shape. This vacuum also allows water, oxygen and nutrient-rich fluids to enter into the disc to allow the spine to heal and relieve the pain. The medical term for this vacuum-like effect is known as negative intradiscal pressure.

Words Defined: Spinal Decompression

A non-surgical therapy that causes the relief of pressure on one or many pinched nerves (neural impingement) of the spinal column.

Patients are fitted with a harness that fits around their hip area as well as a harness that fits around the upper back. Once fitted with the harnesses, the patient lies down on a computerized table, programmed for their specific treatment plan. Each treatment takes about 15 to 25 minutes. The procedure is painless and extremely comfortable.

The typical treatment plan ranges from 18 to 24 sessions over eight to twelve weeks, with most patients experiencing some relief in as little as six sessions

Is Spinal Decompression Safe?

Spinal decompression has proven to be safer and more effective than drugs or surgery. In fact, spinal decompression has in many cases been more effective than chiropractic care when treating severe disc herniations.

The typical way to treat disc bulges and herniations is through medication and injections. The problem with this treatment is that it only masks the pain without addressing the cause of the pain. Although you may feel better, your spine has not been healed and this can lead you to do things that injure your spine further. Additionally, medications are associated with risk and side effects, especially with prolonged use.

Of the medications prescribed for low back pain, the most common are non-steroidal anti-inflammatory drugs, known as NSAIDs. Unlike spinal decompression, these drugs carry significant risks.

Typical side effects of NSAID pills include:

- Nausea
- Stomach pain
- Heartburn
- Dizziness
- Rash
- Constipation
- Diarrhea
- Gas
- Vomiting

More serious side effects of NSAID pills include:

- Allergic reactions
- Bleeding, ulcers
- Perforation of the stomach or intestines
- Liver damage
- Kidney problems, including kidney failure
- Life-threatening bleeding

Even such advice as bed rest can cause problems. These problems include:

- Muscle atrophy
- Heart and lung weakness
- Bone mineral loss
- Blood clots

Of all available options, surgery is the most dangerous, the most expensive and has the lowest success rate. Surgery also has the longest total recovery time and is the most painful treatment option.

The failure rate of surgery for back pain and neck pain is very high. Some 200,000 patients undergo lumbar spine surgery every year. On average, approximately 53 percent of all lumbar spine disc surgeries fail to relieve symptoms.[33]

Then there are the risks for surgery. Risks for back surgery include:

- Failed back surgery syndrome
- Infection
- Nerve damage
- Deterioration of general health
- Post-operative complications

Since spinal decompression does not involve medications or surgery, you will incur none of these risks.

Spinal decompression is not for everyone. For instance, patients who are obese, have metal implants in their spine, or sustained a recent vertebral fracture, are likely not good candidates for this treatment. You will have a complete and thorough medical history and physical exam, as well as review of any X-rays or MRIs of your spine. These tests will help to determine if you are a good candidate for spinal decompression.

CHAPTER 7

Knee Decompression for Knee Pain and Osteoarthritis

Knee pain is something that afflicts millions of people every single day. Whether you have sustained a recent acute injury to your knee joint or you are experiencing chronic pain as the result of regular wear and tear, it can wreak havoc on your overall quality of life. There are many different types of conditions that can lead to knee pain. One of the most common knee problems is osteoarthritis as well as meniscus tears, and ligament and tendon injuries.

Osteoarthritis and "Bone on Bone"

Imagine your knee joint as 2 bones stacked on top of each other forming a hinge. There is cartilage that covers the surface of the joint called articular cartilage. In between these two bones is a joint space (a separation between the two bones) that is incredibly important.

What's So Important About the Joint Space of the Knee?

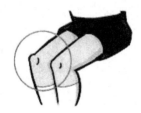

Each of the bones in the knee joint are covered with articular cartilage, which is a tough elastic material, that acts as a shock absorber and allows the knee joint to move with ease. (Another cartilage tissue called the meniscus separates the upper bone (femur) and the lower bone (tibia), divided into two crescent shaped discs located medially and laterally (inner and outer respectively). This cartilage acts as a shock absorber as well as enhances stability.

In a normal knee joint, a **synovium** (synovial membrane) surrounds the knee joint and it produces synovial fluid or **lubrication** that nourishes the surrounding cartilage in the knee. The synovium also protects and supports the joint due to its tough outer layer.

When you have abnormal or excessive stresses on the knee for ANY reason, the cartilage can begin to wear away and break down. **This is called osteoarthritis (OA), which is the most common type of arthritis** (approximately 27 million people are diagnosed with OA in the United States!) This is commonly referred to as the "wear and tear" type of arthritis.

So How Does Osteoarthritis (OA) Damage Your Knee?

Remember that space between the two bones of your knee joint we talked about earlier? The joint space?

When you have OA of the knee:

- The joint space may start to decrease in height and begin to narrow. Some patients get all the way to complete loss of the knee joint space, commonly referred to as "bone on bone."

- Smooth cartilage that normally protects the ends of the knee bones may lose its cushioning effect or become pitted and frayed. Large areas of cartilage may even wear away completely, so the bones scrape painfully over each other.

- Cartilage breakdown may cause the joint to lose its shape, and the bone ends may thicken and form bony spurs.

- The joint is COMPRESSED and fragments of bone or cartilage may float in the joint space, causing further damage and pain.

In addition, as the joint space decreases, what we sometimes see is ligament infolding (ACL, PCL and/or collateral ligaments). This can create adhesions/scar tissue in that knee ligament structure. Knee decompression helps break up that ligamentous scarring and it also, along with the application of Class IV High Intensity Laser, helps to potentially repair the damage to that ligament.

Another benefit of knee decompression is the increase in joint space created between the femur (upper bone) and the tibial plateau (lower bone) in the areas that are compressed. This takes off some of the pressure in the knee, which can help reduce pain and improve function.

The gentle and repetitive motion created during knee decompression treatment also stimulates the production of the patient's own healthy synovial fluid or joint lubrication. This lubrication can also help the knee joint move more freely with less pain.

The traditional way typical doctors treat knee pain is through medication and injections. The problem with this treatment is that it only masks the pain without addressing the cause of the pain. Although you may feel better temporarily, your knee is still compressed and damaged. This can lead you to do things that injure your knee further.

Additionally, medications are associated with risk and side effects, especially with prolonged use.

Of the medications prescribed for knee pain, the most common are non-steroidal anti-inflammatory drugs, known as NSAIDs. Unlike knee decompression, these drugs carry significant risks.

Typical side effects of NSAID pills include:

- Nausea
- Stomach pain
- Heartburn
- Dizziness
- Rash
- Constipation
- Diarrhea
- Gas
- Vomiting

More serious side effects of NSAID pills include:

- Allergic reactions
- Bleeding, ulcers
- Perforation of the stomach or intestines
- Liver damage

- Kidney problems, including kidney failure
- Life-threatening bleeding

Even such advice as bed rest can cause problems. These problems include:

- Muscle atrophy
- Heart and lung weakness
- Bone mineral loss
- Blood clots

Of all available options, knee replacement surgery is potentially the most dangerous and by far the most expensive. Knee replacement surgery also has the longest total recovery time and is the most painful treatment option. Then there are the risks for knee replacement surgery, which include:

- Dislocation
- Infection
- Nerve damage
- Deterioration of general health
- Post-operative complications
- Bone fracture

Since knee decompression does not involve medications or surgery, you will incur none of these risks.

CHAPTER 8

Soft Tissue Therapy That Keeps You Moving!

Soft tissue therapy includes a variety of massage-type treatments of the soft tissue, which includes muscles, connective tissue, ligaments, and tendons. Soft tissue therapy can effectively treat injuries, pain, and dysfunction.

Soft tissue therapy can help with:

- Carpal tunnel syndrome
- Knee and joint pain
- Shin splints
- Back and neck pain
- Plantar fasciitis
- Fibromyalgia
- Tendinitis

- Groin pulls
- Frozen shoulder

Benefits of Soft Tissue Therapy

Soft tissue therapy is effective in alleviating many symptoms associated with those medical conditions listed above. It can improve the performance of your muscles and joints. It can also improve range of motion and alleviate the pain and stiffness secondary to arthritis, back and neck pain and neuropathy.

Trigger Point Therapy

Trigger points are those tender "knots" you feel when you or someone rubs a sore spot. Our physical therapists will apply pressure to trigger points to relieve pain and dysfunction in other parts of the body – this is called trigger point therapy.

There are two basic types of trigger points: active and latent.

- Active trigger points cause muscular pain and transfer pain to other areas of the body when your chiropractor applies pressure. For example, pressing on a trigger point between your shoulders may send shooting pain down your arm.

• Latent trigger points do not refer pain to other areas of the body, and cause stiffness in the joints and restricted range of motion.

Trigger points develop due to several causes, including birth trauma, an injury sustained in a fall or accident, poor posture, or overexertion.

After several treatments of trigger point therapy, the swelling and stiffness of muscular pain is reduced, range of motion is increased, tension is relieved, and circulation, flexibility and coordination are improved.

Cross Friction Massage

Soft tissues can become stressed beyond their limits, resulting in small, microscopic tears. When these tears occur, the body responds by causing inflammation, which helps in the role of healing.

However, too much inflammation can form scar tissue.

Continuing to use the muscle as it is torn can increase the chance of more scarring. Scar tissue is tough and decreases mobility and elasticity. This results in loss of function, resulting in more tearing and inflammation, resulting in more scar tissue... a vicious cycle.

For cross friction massage, your physical therapist will apply his fingers directly over the tissue involved. The key here is for the massage to be opposite the direction of the tissue fibers. This "transverse friction" massage keeps adhesions and scar tissue from forming. It also results in improved range of motion and less pain.

Cross friction massage is a highly effective treatment for injuries to the muscles, tendons, and ligaments caused by micro-tears. Cross friction creates heat, which helps to mobilize adhesions (bands of scar tissue) between fascial layers, muscles, and other soft tissues. This heat helps to promote healing.

Knee injuries are extremely common, but the healing process can be quite frustrating. In a 2009 study, bilateral knee injuries were treated with cross friction massage one week following injury. Fifty-one participants received between nine and 30 treatments. After four weeks of cross friction massage, the knees were stronger, less stiff and could absorb more energy.[34]

Myofascial Release Therapy

Myofascial release is a stretching technique used by some physical therapists to treat soft tissue problems. To understand what it is and how it works, you first need to know a few things about fascia.

Fascia is a thin tissue that covers the muscles and every fiber within each muscle. This means that when you stretch your muscles, you are really stretching your muscles and your fascia.

When muscle fibers are injured, the fibers and the fascia surrounding it become short and tight. This uneven stress can cause pain and other symptoms. Myofascial release treats these symptoms by releasing the uneven tightness in injured fascia.

The stretching is determined by our physical therapist as he feels what each stretch does to your body. The feedback he receives helps him decide how much force to use, the direction of the stretch, and how long to stretch.

Our physical therapists will find areas of tightness and then apply a light stretch. Once your muscle and fascia have relaxed, he will increase the stretch. This process is repeated until the area is fully relaxed. Then, the next affected area is stretched.

One area that myofascial release therapy holds great promise is in the treatment of scoliosis, which is an abnormal curvature of the spine. A 2008 case study of an 18-year-old female subject observed her progress as she underwent six weeks of myofascial release therapy. The subject received treatment consisting of two sessions each week for 60 minutes. Pain, pulmonary function and quality of life were measured at predetermined intervals.

The subject improved with pain levels, trunk rotation, posture, quality of life, and pulmonary function.[35]

Which type of soft tissue therapy is right for you? Our team will evaluate what type of muscle work you may need and administer the appropriate treatments as part of the Restore-Care™ protocol. These treatments work together to provide better circulation, pain relief and range of motion in a shorter amount of time than any one modality can deliver on its own.

CHAPTER 9

Good Health Starts with Good Nutrition

Getting regular exercise, dealing with stress in healthy ways, and eating a diet rich in plant-based whole foods is a great start toward achieving good health. But no matter how well you stick to these tips, you are always at risk for your body to be damaged at the cellular level. Environmental factors play a huge part in this damage by introducing free radicals into our bodies.

What Are Free Radicals?

Free radicals form in the human body when an electron in an atom becomes unpaired and searches for another electron to pair with. It may sounds like an insignificant event, but this search for another unpaired atom causes damage to our cells and a chain reaction of more free radical creation.

Daily life exposes us to free radicals all the time, from the foods we eat and the air we breathe. Free radicals cause illness and contribute to the aging process. They have a negative impact on how we look and feel. Free radicals occur in everyday life but are made worse by:

- Eating a diet full of processed foods and produce treated with chemicals
- Smoking
- Using drugs
- Failure to deal correctly with stress
- Excessive sun exposure
- Pollution

Free radical damage can lead to:

- Cancer
- Heart Disease
- Diabetes
- Arthritis
- Autoimmune diseases

One thing we can do to fight free radicals is to get more antioxidants in our diet. Antioxidants are vitamins, minerals, and other nutrients that protect the body and fight off free radicals. They give free radicals an electron to pair with before the stray electrons can damage our cells. Some examples of antioxidants are beta carotene, vitamin C, and vitamin E. These vitamins help strengthen the immune system, too. Plus, they're readily available in many plant-based foods which we should consume more of, anyway!

Beta Carotene

Beta carotene is one of a group of red, orange, and yellow pigments called carotenoids. Beta carotene and other carotenoids provide approximately 50% of the Vitamin A needed in our daily diet.[36]

Beta carotene is a substance the body converts into Vitamin A. It's a powerful antioxidant that also helps protect the cells and boost the immune system. Sources of this important nutrient include:

- Carrots
- Pumpkins
- Sweet Potatoes
- Spinach
- Collards
- Kale
- Turnip greens
- Beet greens
- Winter squash
- Cabbage

If you would rather get your vitamin A straight-up instead of through the beta carotene conversion, eat more:

- Beef
- Broccoli
- Cantaloupe
- Apricots
- Liver
- Milk
- Butter
- Cheese
- Whole eggs

Vitamin C

When your mom told you to drink orange juice to get over a cold faster, she was right! Vitamin C is another antioxidant that strengthens the immune system. It's vital to the growth and repair of skin, blood vessels, ligaments, and tendons. It is also involved with healing wounds and forming scar tissue.

Plus, vitamin C is important for the formation of collagen, which holds your body's cells together. And, it plays an important role in maintaining oral and eye health.

Many fruits are excellent sources of vitamin C, including:

- Cantaloupe
- Citrus fruits
- Kiwi
- Mango
- Guava
- Papaya
- Pineapple

- Berries
- Watermelon

You can get vitamin C from vegetables too, like cruciferous veggies (broccoli, cauliflower, and Brussels sprouts), peppers, leafy greens, potatoes, tomatoes, and squash.

Vitamin E

The third antioxidant we're concerned about is vitamin E. This nutrient helps widen blood vessels and keeps blood from clotting inside them. Foods that are high in vitamin E will also protect your skin from ultraviolet light, which is a major cause of free radical formation in the body.

Excellent sources of vitamin E include:

- Spinach
- Chard
- Turnip greens
- Mustard greens
- Cayenne pepper
- Asparagus
- Bell peppers

- Eggs
- Nuts and seeds
- Meats
- Olive oil
- Whole grains

Nutrition

Eating a well-balanced diet should provide essential nutrients, but there are some situations that definitely call for adding in supplements. When your diet isn't properly balanced, it doesn't contain adequate amounts of certain nutrients. In this case, supplements may be absolutely necessary.

In order for our body to use food to repair and create cells and tissues, it needs the proper tools. The following nutrients are extremely important to maintain a healthy body. And just like the majority of antioxidant sources, these nutrients are often found in abundance in plant-sourced foods.

Magnesium is not only an essential nutrient, but is responsible for a vast variety of healthy body functions. It also is the most deficient mineral in the Standard American Diet because it can be difficult to meet the daily requirements just from food. Less than 30% of U.S. adults consume the Recommended Daily Allowance of magnesium. And nearly 20% get only half of the magnesium they need daily to remain healthy.[37]

To make sure you get enough magnesium in your diet, eat plenty of whole grains, legumes, vegetables, nuts, seeds, and seafood.

Calcium is the most abundant mineral in your body. It is responsible for strong teeth and bones, as well as proper function of blood vessels, nerve communication, and muscles. Many Americans suffer from a deficiency in calcium. We lose calcium each day through our skin, nails, hair, sweat, and waste.

To make sure you get enough calcium in your diet, make sure you consume dairy products, broccoli, kale, Chinese cabbage, and salmon regularly. Depending on your diet and age, your doctor might recommend a calcium supplement.

Iron is important for the production of hemoglobin (found in red blood cells) and myoglobin (found in muscles). These proteins carry and store oxygen throughout the body. When you don't have enough iron in your body you feel tired, weak, and unable to focus. Few people ever have too much iron in the body, but this rare condition is toxic.

Excellent sources of iron include red meat, liver, egg yolks, leafy green veggies, dried fruits, shellfish, beans, lentils, and artichokes. Pairing iron-rich foods with vitamin C-rich foods will help your body absorb the iron better.[38]

Iron deficiency can affect anyone, but it is extremely common among women of childbearing age. Your chiropractor can help you adjust your diet or recommend an iron supplement when necessary.

Vitamin D helps our bodies in the absorption of calcium. Vitamin D also increases bone density and helps prevent bone fractures. Plus, calcium helps regulate the immune system and protects against some types of cancer.

Humans can synthesize their own vitamin D – all it takes is a little sunshine. If you spend a little time in the sun each day, it is unlikely you will be deficient in vitamin D.

People in warm climates rarely have vitamin D problems – it's our neighbors to the north who tend to hibernate through cold, cloudy winters who suffer. If you live far north of the equator, all it really takes is exposing your skin to the sun for about 20 minutes per day (or a little bit longer for older or dark-skinned people) prior to applying sunscreen on most summer days. If you do this, your body will probably synthesize enough vitamin D to last the whole year.[39]

Folic acid is a B vitamin. It helps your body make new cells, repair DNA, and prevent Alzheimer's, anemia, and some forms of cancer.

It is extremely important for pregnant women to get enough folic acid not only while pregnant, but prior to pregnancy too. One of the first stages of pregnancy includes the development of the brain and spinal cord, so getting enough folic acid during this process is vital to proper fetal development. Insufficient folic acid has been linked to birth defects including spina bifida and anencephaly.

Veggies and citrus fruits are the best sources of folic acid. Eat plenty of dark leafy greens, asparagus, broccoli, beans, citrus fruits, peas, lentils, avocado, seeds and nuts, carrots, and squash.

Eating a healthy, well-balanced diet can provide you with a strong, energetic, efficient, healthy body. The best way to know if you are getting all the elements that make up a fully functioning healthy body is to discuss your diet with your chiropractor or health care professional. Together, you can ensure that you are providing the optimum fuel to your body.

Your body is designed to heal itself. The nervous system is what controls your immune system. If you're run down, your body is less able to cope with germs and infections. This is when we tend to experience illness or pain. If your nervous system is strong and healthy, your body can deal with injuries and germs better. One of our main areas of focus here at **Relief Source** is helping you maintain a strong and healthy nervous system, resulting in a healthy body and lifestyle.

CHAPTER 10

Getting Back to the Basics of Wellness

For a moment, think back to when you were a kid. Chances are that back in elementary school, you had boundless energy. The days were long but it didn't matter – you could probably run around the neighborhood with your friends with hardly a thought of food, pain, or fatigue.

Now maybe you have kids or grandkids, and you watch them go at playtime for hours without a pause – and it's exhausting! We joke about bottling all that energy. We get nostalgic about feeling limitless and free, but not enough of us know that there really is a way to regain some of those powerful feelings again.

Wellness is very personal and means different things to different people in terms of preferences and outcomes.

- If you have debilitating back pain, you might feel powerful again if you could get through the day without taking prescription painkillers and suffering through their side effects.

- If your knee arthritis restricts your daily physical activities, you might feel powerful again if you could go for a hike again, or even just do your normal daily activities without it resulting in days of excruciating joint pain.

- If you suffer from peripheral neuropathy, you might feel powerful again if you could regain sensation in your fingertips again and take up the activities and hobbies you left behind years ago.

Getting older isn't always easy – but remember that we are lucky to have made it this far!

So what will it take for you to get out of pain and feel energetic and powerful again? Every person presents their own set of symptoms, conditions, and function limits. Plus, each person has their own set of goals that will make them feel healthy and happy.

As we discussed in prior chapters, we offer multiple healing modalities as part of our comprehensive Restore-Care™ protocol that patients with chronic pain find to be beneficial. We also counsel our patients who are interested in learning about the importance of eating a well-balanced diet.

Good nutrition should be considered the cornerstone of any wellness plan. The food you use to fuel your body will make a huge difference when your cells need to repair and regenerate themselves. We promote a diet that's big on unprocessed foods, fruits, vegetables, whole grains, and lean protein. Eating like this gives your body the vitamins, minerals, and antioxidants it needs to stay strong and healthy.

What Should I Do if I Suspect That I Have Peripheral Neuropathy or Chronic Back, Knee or Joint Pain?

The National Institutes of Neurological Disorders and Stroke says that peripheral neuropathy affects roughly 24 million Americans.[40] It's a very common condition among people in certain populations, such as diabetics, cancer patients, and those taking statin medications to lower their cholesterol. Therefore, it's important to know that if you do have peripheral neuropathy, you are certainly not alone.

Severe back and knee arthritis typically show structurally damaged tissues on X-ray or MRI. It's likely if you have been suffering for some time, this test may have already been performed, revealing these issues.

While the early stages of back, knee or nerve symptoms may seem to be just minor irritations, early diagnosis of these conditions can potentially prevent the condition from becoming worse. Talk to your doctor right away to diagnose and determine the cause of your chronic pain. There could be ways to change your medical treatment plan that can reduce your symptoms.

We also strongly recommend visiting one of our Relief Source Spine & Joint Rehab Centers as soon as you can. They will be able to determine if you're a good candidate for their Restore-Care™ treatment protocol that can reduce or even eliminate the pain, numbness, and tingling associated with chronic back and neck pain, chronic knee pain and peripheral neuropathy. They also have non-surgical protocols for shoulder, hip, elbow, ankle/foot and many other musculoskeletal conditions. There is no reason to wait until the problem becomes worse – as soon as you suspect that something is wrong, seek professional help. It's the best way to ensure your health and wellness for many years to come.

CHAPTER 11

Success Stories

"Before starting treatments with Dr. Stephen Lembo with Spinal Decompression, for 2 years I'd had MRIs, CAT Scans, Acupuncture, and physical therapy before and after my spinal surgery. I was diagnosed with spinal stenosis, herniated and bulging discs, degenerative disc disease and sciatic pain over the left hip and leg. My problem caused difficulty walking, balancing, standing, and pain and tightness in my back so much that I had to walk with the support of a cane. I noticed an ad in Newsday which listed all of my existing problems and claimed a "new treatment without surgery. My attitude was why not? I had tried everything else with only temporary relief. I called and made an appointment for a consultation. All my questions and concerns were answered. I was shown the Spinal Decompression technology with an explanation of how it works. I was accepted as a candidate and started care. In my profession I am fully aware that "Tender Loving Care" goes a long way in the healing process. Dr. Lembo and his staff provided that and made the entire experience comfortable, enjoyable, and encouraging. For this I am grateful. I finished my Spinal Decompression treatment in six short weeks. I can now walk and stand WITHOUT THE CANE. I rejoined my Senior Citizen's Singing and Dancing Performance Group and I'm back on tour! Thanks to Dr. Lembo and his staff **Ain't No Stoppin' Me Now**!"

Gloria E.
Retired Registered Nurse
Age 75

"I was suffering with numbness, tingling and pain in both hands for over 2 years prior to starting Dr. Lembo's laser program. My arms and hands would get numb especially while sleeping. Since starting treatment I have had much less numbness and I've been sleeping better at night. The friendliness and *professionalism displayed by Dr. Lembo and his staff is unmatched by any other office I've EVER been in."*

Vincent C.
49 years old

"It has now been 4 months since I finished my laser therapy treatment with you and I am so pleased. I came in suffering from a very painful left elbow often called Tennis or Golf elbow. After each treatment I felt less pain even though I continued to play golf regularly. I have no pain or soreness in that elbow since the treatment and am therefore pleased to recommend the laser treatment. I also want to praise the entire staff who made every visit a pleasurable experience. I have been telling all of my friends about them!"

Peter S.

"When I first started seeing Dr. Lembo I had constant pain in my wrists that impaired me from doing basic everyday things like picking up my younger daughter, and I wasn't prepared to stop doing that at any cost. Through therapy, I felt better and better each week

until it wasn't a problem anymore...I know I'm in good hands."

Arleen S.
Age 32

"I started with pain, numbness, tingling in my right hand and a burning sensation in my left hand. Dr. Lembo's treatments have improved my symptoms 50% in both hands, giving me the ability to sleep better at night and I'm less bothered during the day by pain and numbness. Dr. Lembo and staff are very caring. Thank You so much!"

Richard T.
77 years old

"For over 30 years, I have woken up almost every morning with annoying numbness and tingling in my hands. I have tried various treatments over the years, but nothing ever helped. Prior to starting treatments with Dr. Lembo, I must admit I was a skeptic because I've has this condition for so long and no other doctor has been able to help me...I was afraid I might be a "hopeless case". To my surprise and delight, his treatments really worked – and fast. **It's a miracle that after only 12 treatments, I woke up without that annoying numbness in my hands for the first time in 30 years!** I owe it all to Dr. Lembo and his Carpal Tunnel Relief Program."

Gloria C.

Age 63

"It wasn't very long ago that I came to you suffering from a knee injury, unable to bend my knee and pain with every step. An orthopedic surgeon diagnosed bone-on bone, recommended cortisone injections or perhaps a knee replacement. Your confidence in the healing properties in the new high power deep tissue laser therapy convinced me to try it. After only three treatments I was able to bend the knee without much pain! Today, after five treatments, I can bend the knee almost pain free!! And, each step is no longer agony. I am so grateful to you and your staff and look forward to continuing the full course of treatment and a pain free knee!"

Joan H.

"Before starting care I suffered with shooting tingling in my left hand and fingers that traveled up my forearm. After 6 months of suffering, I consulted with Dr. Lembo about his Laser Program. He determined I was a good candidate and I started care. Now after only 5 short weeks my condition has improved at least 90%. The program really works and I highly recommend Dr. Lembo's program to anyone, of <u>any age</u> suffering with carpal tunnel. Thanks a million Doc!"

Ignazio C.
Age 80

"Before starting Dr. Lembo's Laser Program, I was in great pain and I couldn't use my right hand for everyday things like writing, vacuuming and doing minor chores around the house. I'm happy to say I am very pleased with the treatment and care that was given to me by Dr. Lembo and his staff and would gladly come back for any future treatment needs!"

Dolores M.
Age 72

"I just wanted to send you this thank you regarding the benefits of laser therapy. This is a life savior from pain relief. Miraculously with the first treatment amazing the relief has been immediate and improved with each treatment. Thank God no more pain, instead of tears I smile from ear to ear. Thank you."

Marcia W.

"I would like to thank you for introducing me to his new laser treatment. I came in with a lot of pain in my neck, however the laser treatment has taken the pain away. I am slowly going back to training the way I used to. Thanks."

Frank H.

"My left wrist and forearm had shooting pains and would get numb and tingling whenever my left hand was elevated for a couple of minutes. When I first started treatment with Dr. Lembo, I was very impressed with the fact that I was never left waiting. If my appointment was for 10 AM or 6 PM I was in for treatment at that time. The staff is very efficient and friendly. After my treatments with Dr. Lembo's Laser program, my wrist no longer bothers me. I'm glad I answered the ad in Newsday. Thank you Dr. Lembo!"

Charles C.
Age 67

"I had severe pain and tingling in my right hand to the point where it kept me awake at night. I had tried everything – gloves, creams, exercises and anything anyone told me would help. Nothing did. However, your Laser treatments have given me back the use of my hand. I am now able to do my quilting again and normal everyday things that people take for granted. It has been a pleasure to have known Dr. Lembo and his wonderful staff. I can't thank you all enough for helping me return to my normal day-to-day living."

Justine P.
Age 85

"I want to thank you for giving me the opportunity to try the Laser Therapy Treatment. Your enthusiasm for this treatment convinced me to give it a try, after one treatment on my hip I felt so little pain that it was not necessary to take my painkillers. I have not taken any medication for five days now, and still feeling very good, I am continuing this treatment and urge you to give it a try."

Antonia C.

"The first time I tried the laser treatment it was a little warm at first and my wrist felt amazing. After a past fracture I have been unable to do too much with my wrist and now since the laser treatment I am able to do everything. I recommend anyone try this treatment."

Jeremy B.

"The one benefit I value most that I received from Dr. Lembo is the instant and lasting relief I get at each visit. Dr. Lembo's treatments on my neck has greatly reduced my tension headaches, which has made my life much easier. In addition, the treatments on my wrist have improved my carpal tunnel syndrome and **I have cancelled plans for surgery on my hand.**

Treatments on my back has eased the pain I felt at work and has made me more comfortable. My overall feeling toward the practice is EXCELLENT!"

Mark B.

Age 53

"*After only 3 treatments using the laser, the changes in my mobility and flexibility in my lower back has greatly improved. The other change that has made a difference is the decrease in inflammation, which in turn reduces my pain level. My thanks for integrating laser into your practice.*"

Debra R.

"*I was in extreme pain in the wrist area of my right hand. I was using Celebrex 2x daily, and a wrist brace at night.... I don't need any of these aids any more. My wrist feels normal again. I'm not afraid to use my right hand like I used to- it's a wonderful feeling! I can't wait to return to my yard work! Thank you, Dr. Lembo!*"

Lucy S.

Age 49

"After my wrist fracture wasn't healing well and there was constant swelling and inflammation, I came to start using laser therapy. Three weeks later I feel much, much better at 70%. Thanks for your help."

Ana H

"As a carpenter, the abuse to my hands is there every day. Since working with Dr. Lembo, I got relief from the pain and numbness. The treatments are relaxing and painless."

Joseph B.
Age 46

"After injuring my back at the gym over 8 months ago, I had suffered with a disc herniation that pressed on my nerve and caused pain. After 7 months of non-stop physical therapy, massage and chiropractic care nothing helped to relieve the pain. The next step my doctor recommended was spinal injections, which I wasn't thrilled about. But after learning more about Spinal Decompression, I set up a consultation to discuss my condition with Dr. Lembo. I decided to give it a try. Now, after only 6 weeks, my treatments have ended and I haven't had any pain. I started back at the gym and I feel GREAT! Post MRI shows NO EVIDENCE of disc herniation after Dr. Lembo's Spinal Decompression Program. This result is truly amazing and documented!"

Michele G.
Age 42

"Before I was a patient with Dr. Lembo, I was taking pain medication 2-3 times daily (Vicodin) and even with that I still had severe pain. I own my own business and I was going to have to sell it. I could not take walks with my family or play with my kids. Since my treatments with Dr. Lembo and his Spinal Decompression my life has completely changed. Now I can do almost anything I want with very little pain and since I am still improving and getting treatments I think there is a very good chance that I will be 100% better by the time I am done. Just a note: The entire staff is amazingly friendly and helpful. They have given me my life back the way it was!"

Mike J.
Age 49

"Prior to starting care with Dr. Lembo's Spinal Decompression program, I had been suffering with chronic back pain for over 37 years. The severity of my pain has varied over the years and I was looking for a solution to my back pain that had the ability to fix the disc. I was no longer interested in masking the pain with all those other traditional treatments most doctors recommend. Since starting Spinal Decompression with Dr. Lembo, I'm excited to say that this is the best I've felt in years. I only wish this technology was around when I first hurt my back 37 years ago! I am looking forward to living my next 37+ years pain- free and doing everything I enjoy. I would recommend Dr. Lembo to anyone suffering with a low back disc problem. He had shown a genuine concern for my well-being and the entire staff has been outstanding from day one."

Shan B.
Age 61

"Prior to coming in, I had researched Decompression technology and decided to consult with Dr. Lembo to see if it had a chance to help my condition. I suffered with chronic back problems including disc herniations for many years, tried a variety of different treatments and I have lived with intermittent problems for years that included tingling, sharp, shooting and burning symptoms. I finished treatment after 6 weeks, and I would say that I am considerably better than before I started treatment. I would recommend Dr. Lembo and this procedure to anyone with chronic back pain from herniated discs in the low back. The entire process, from evaluation through treatment has been very positive; a very friendly environment to come and get well!"

Doug P.
Age 60

"Before starting Spinal Decompression treatments with Dr. Lembo, I was suffering for over 10 months with low back pain and sciatica from 5 bulging and degenerative discs in my low back. The pain became so severe that it kept me from working for approximately 7 to 8 months. I went to the neurologist, orthopedist, internal medicine doctor, chiropractor, acupuncture, cardiologist, pain management and even consulted with a neurosurgeon. I desperately wanted to avoid surgery but I had reached the end of doctors to see. That's when I called for one of Dr. Lembo's back pain reports in the mail. I read the entire report from front to back and I immediately called for my free consultation. When Dr. Lembo accepted my case, I was thrilled to have a real chance to feel better again. I knew this was my last resort and it was. Now after only 20 treatments, I feel 200% better than I did only 5 weeks ago. Not only that, Dr. Lembo and his entire staff are, in one word...excellent! For anyone looking for a real legitimate, no gimmicks treatment for back pain, this is it!

Irwin L.
Age 78

"I had had chronic back pain for 18 years due to bulging and degenerative discs. Prior to coming in for my consultation I was VERY SKEPTICAL that there was anything out there that could help me. I had tried chiropractic, acupuncture and Advil over the years and none of that was able to help my back problem. I was concerned because my condition was progressively getting worse over the last 2 years and I started missing some time from work. I wasn't even able to play a round of golf without pain. More importantly, my two children are very active, I coach my son's little league team and I was concerned about missing out on spending quality time with them. One day while reading Newsday, I saw one of Dr. Lembo's ads about a new treatment for disc problems. With nothing to lose, I ordered his free report. The report gave me some hope that it might help my condition but I was skeptical because it almost sounded too good to be true. But I called anyway and scheduled my consultation. I was a bit apprehensive coming in that first time, but Dr. Lembo and his entire staff made my whole experience very comfortable. He was very thorough in his evaluation and had me come back for

a second visit to go over the details of my condition. When Dr. Lembo determined that I was a good candidate for Spinal Decompression, I was excited to start treatments. Now after 5 weeks my treatments are coming to an end and I'm happy to report I feel 100% better. And my function has returned the way I had hoped. More importantly, for the first time in 18 years, I feel like I'm being healed for life. My whole experience with Spinal Decompression has made me very happy and Dr. Lembo's dedication to helping me get well is just fantastic. And by the way, last week at my son's little league practice, I was able to pitch over 400 balls (at over 45 miles per hour) to the kids... without any problem...pain free! I'm living proof that in only 5 short weeks, Dr. Lembo's Program can change your life!"

Darren E.
Age 46

"I was suffering with lower back pain for years. I tried spinal injections, went through TWO BACK OPERATIONS...tried physical therapy, chiropractic and exercise. Nothing helped. I was having a hard

time walking even short distances without my cane. After 5 short weeks of treatment, I can now walk for extended distances without pain...and without my cane! Having tried everything, Dr. Lembo's Spinal Decompression treatment program is the only treatment that has me up and walking. I thank God... and recommend Dr. Lembo without hesitation to anyone of any age suffering with severe back pain to try his program."

Helen M.

Age 81

*"When I first came to Dr. Steve Lembo, I could barely walk or function properly...**I had <u>two</u> herniated discs, sciatica and a compressed nerve** that affected my lower back and left leg. I was in constant pain all the time. My job requires me to be on my feet 12 to 13 hours a day which made things even more difficult for me day by day. Searching for a solution, I met with Dr. Lembo. He felt I was a good candidate for his procedures and started treatment with his Spinal Decompression program. Let me just say that after only 5 weeks, I'm a new man! Now work is MUCH*

THE DEFINITIVE GUIDE TO BACK, JOINT, AND NERVE PAIN RELIEF!

easier and **going up and down the stairs at least 40 times a day is a piece of cake.** I recommend this procedure to anyone who does not want to go the surgical route. Dr. Lembo has changed the quality of my life."

John C.
Age 53

"Before my start with Dr. Lembo and the Spinal Decompression treatment, I was so immersed and overwhelmed by the pain caused due to my low back condition (2 disc herniations, 2 disc bulges and degenerated discs), that I couldn't see or think straight. I couldn't even sleep through the night without the terrible pain waking me up. People can't imagine how lack of sleep can control your very existence. I was beginning to feel like a very unproductive human being and all that mattered to me was to find a solution to my discomfort so I could get my life back together again. I read Dr. Lembo's free report, called his office and made an appointment. I didn't know what to expect by coming in that first day. Of course I was skeptical and unsure *of the success of the treatment since the technology was new to me. Most people are skeptical of the unknown. But after Dr. Lembo was able to explain to me what the problem was and how the technology works to FIX the problem, it made complete sense to me and I knew this was something new and different that I had to try. Now 6 weeks later, as my treatments are coming to an end, I once again feel like a member of the human race. What's more, I can sleep through the night for the first time in months! I can honestly say that Dr. Lembo has changed my life for the better. I'm looking forward to getting back to work...feeling like a contributing member of society. Even more importantly, friends and family are commenting about how good I look and how positive my attitude and energy is now compared to before treatment with Spinal Decompression started. Thank you, Dr. Lembo. I appreciate all your help more than you can imagine!"*

Frank C.
Age 64

"I tried everything over the years, I'm pain-free after one laser treatment! It's a miracle. My first treatment I went from 0% to 70% with no more pain in my knee. I can stand up better and my walking is much better. Thank You!"

Mamie

"Before starting here, I was in pain for almost two years. Back and leg pain. I tried Chiropractors, all kinds of Medical Doctors, physical therapy for one year and two epidurals. Nothing helped me. Now, after treatments with Dr. Lembo and Spinal Decompression, I can lead a normal life. The first benefit for me is not constantly thinking about pain... having a bright future...doing the things I want to do. Secondly, getting a good night's sleep is wonderful. I am grateful to Dr. Lembo and his program. Many Thanks!"

Carolyn M.
Age 61

"Before being treated by Dr. Lembo with Spinal Decompression, I had chronic pain in my lower back and both legs. I could not take a step, or sit down without pain. A few years ago before retiring, I started to have pain in my right leg and lower back. I tried physical therapy but after months of that the pain did not go away...in fact the pain got worse and it forced me to retire. At that point I started with a new therapist, and after another 2 months of therapy it seemed as if there was nothing anyone could do for me. At that time my life had changed, I felt as if I was handicapped and I was thinking...what am I going to do now? My wife saw an ad in Newsday about Dr. Stephen Lembo. It listed all of the pain that I had. I thought this is too good to be true, but my wife said "How would you know if you don't call and find out?" By this time I had used deep penetrating pain relievers, every kind of pain medication that my system would tolerate, but I still had pain, so I made the call to Dr. Stephen Lembo's office. That was the best decision I could have made. From the first interview I was confident that Dr. Lembo could help. After a week, I started to feel better, and after 5 weeks, I was able

to do a stress test which in itself was strenuous, **I was able to walk on a treadmill at 5.6 miles per hour for 12 minutes WITHOUT PAIN.** Although I still have some dull pain, it's nothing that I can't live with and since I'm still being treated and cared for by Dr. Lembo and his staff, I feel that I will be completely healed in a very short period of time. I'm elated with the progress I've made with this procedure."

Paul K.

Age 71

"For the past few years I have suffered from Morton's Neuroma. An orthopedic gave me three cortisone injections years ago, but they only provided relief while the topical analgesic was active. I knew the next step was surgery....but it's in both feet, and when can I find the time to be off my feet? Never. Plus, there was no guarantee. So, I've suffered terribly, with burning, searing pain, usually about a half hour after I start walking. I usually take off my shoes for about ten minutes, and then I'm fine. For another little while, until I have to do it again. After the FIRST laser treatment (6 mins on each foot), I haven't had the issue again. I felt a bit of it coming on a day or so ago, but it hasn't gotten to the painful stage. Therefore, I want to continue treatment until I forget I ever even had it. This condition interfered with my usual active, energetic life. Now, that I've discovered this miraculous, painless, amazing treatment, I know I'll never suffer again!!! Thank you for introducing it to me. It's worth the cost!! (Less than surgery, quicker, no recovery time, and no loss of wages for missed work...etc.) It's like a magic wand that costs just a bit but makes a phenomenal difference! I'm GRATEFUL!"

Jana W.

"Before I became a patient of Dr. Lembo's in June, I was suffering with a great deal of pain in my lower back. The pain traveled down the right side of my leg below my knee. I could not sit without experiencing pain. I received spinal decompression treatments – following Dr. Lembo's program. In time, I was able to resume my normal activities – playing tennis and golf. And I'm also now enjoying a normal social life with my wife. I found Dr. Lembo and his staff to be caring, supportive, concerned and accommodating.

They were very interested in my welfare. I am very appreciative that they enabled me to "get my life back."

Peter R.
Age 63

"I would like to thank you for recommending the laser treatment for my neck pain. I originally came to you wanting to have MUA (Manipulation under Anesthesia), which is an invasive procedure. When you recommended the laser treatment instead, I must admit that I was apprehensive. But was I wrong!!! Thank you for your advice and most caring treatment."

Frank Q.

"If anyone in this group is suffering with lower back pain and/or leg pain from bulging herniated or slipped disc I have to let you in on what I did to finally get my problem fixed.....no drugs.......no injections.... no surgery! I could hardly walk with the pain in my lower back and down my right leg - could not sleep - only comfort was sitting down. I finally decided to

see an Orthopedic Doctor who ordered an MRI which showed 5 severely herniated bulging discs in my lower back - leaning on a nerve and shooting pain down my right leg - he gave me a prednisone pack that you have to wean yourself off of and told me if that didn't relieve my pain I would need injections and if that didn't work then I'd have to have surgery. I didn't know what to do as my activities were very limited and I would have done anything to avoid surgery. I tried the prednisone pack and it gave me temporary relief but the pain came back. Soon after, I heard of this chiropractor (Dr. Lembo) near my job that has a non-surgical Spinal Decompression machine. I feel it is a miracle how I got my life back. I had about 24 sessions and I would say after the 5th one - I started feeling a big difference and this is a permanent fix. I am truly a new person. I highly recommend Dr. Lembo to anyone suffering with low back disc problems - He is one of the 1st offices on Long Island to offer this procedure and has the most experience in how to work this technology to get the best results."

Connie P.
Age 60

"Prior to starting Spinal Decompression treatment with Dr. Lembo, I had severe low back pain as well as severe pain in my right thigh. The pain started over 5 months ago and resulted in limitations of all activities including running around with the kids, walking my dog, any forward bending and even sitting for long periods of time. I had two disc herniations that produced pain that was sharp, shooting, stabbing and achy. The pain became so severe that I sought out various types of treatment... physical therapy, epidural injections, prescription medication, and cortisone injections. I was frustrated and a bit discouraged to find that these approached did not provide a solution for my pain and I became concerned that I may need surgery. Reading Newsday one morning, I saw an ad and called the 1-800 # to get the free report on back pain. I drove to the office feeling very skeptical that the treatment would be able to fix my problem especially after trying almost everything that was out there. But I knew I had absolutely nothing to lose except 30 minutes of my time. Once I arrived at the office, I immediately felt I was in a very professional environment where both Dr. Lembo and his staff were *not only professional, but personable as well. After the consultation, examination and review of my MRI, I came back for a second visit when Dr. Lembo was able to explain my problem, why the other treatments I tried didn't work for healing my disc problems and how Spinal Decompression works. I started treatment and I quickly saw results. By only the 4th or 5th visit, the treatment began to relieve much of the spasm that was occurring in my right leg, enabling me to walk normally. After 4 weeks, neither my back nor my leg hurt. Now in my last few weeks of treatment, all that's left is some tightness in my low back, but not pain! I now have the ability to perform normal everyday tasks."*

Derrick W.
Age 43

"I came here with BONE ON BONE, lots of knee pain and very little mobility. Now after 12 sessions, I'm walking up stairs again, playing golf, able to get up from a chair with comfort, sleeping through the night and taking vacations again. I'm just a little stiff in the morning but when you consider Bone on Bone...what

I had before to where I am now – IT'S AMAZING. ABSOLUTELY AMAZING! I highly recommend you give it a try. You'll be a lot happier!"

John P.
Age 73
Mt. Sinai, NY

The Honest Truth, I Was Skeptical This Would Work For Me...
But Now At Age 79, I Can Do <u>Anything</u> I Want WITHOUT Pain...!

"About 4 months ago, my low back and right leg pain got to the point where the pain was so severe, I checked myself into the Emergency Room at the hospital. They gave me strong prescription pain pills, which didn't help with the pain one bit. Soon after, I went to my medical doctor and he gave me different pills to try but again, the medication did not help my pain. My situation was very bad. My pain level was a 10 out of 10. I couldn't lie down because the pain was so severe and I wasn't able to sleep for several months. I was tired and exhausted. I was also unable

to even sit down without intense pain so I had to eat breakfast, lunch and dinner STANDING UP! Then one day, my wife was on the computer, I think Facebook, and she learned about Relief Source and what they were doing to help severe back pain patients like me get out of pain and fixed. TO TELL YOU THE HONEST TRUTH...I WAS SKEPTICAL. But with nothing to lose, I scheduled my free consultation to see if he could help. After the doctor did his evaluation and MRI review, he determined I was a good candidate for his program of Warm Laser with Spinal Decompression and he accepted my case for treatment. THE DECISION I MADE TO START CARE WAS THE BEST DECISION I MADE! The pain started to improve quickly, (after the first few visits), and then each week thereafter, more and more improvement. My back and leg pain that was once so severe and crippling was now getting better and better! I was able to sit for longer periods of time without pain and FINALLY I could sleep through the night without the pain waking me up. NOW, THE PAIN IS AT A ZERO. I feel great, actually wonderful, and I can now, at age 79 do anything I want to do without limits! I would absolutely recommend Relief

Source to my family and friends. My sister lives in South Carolina but I wish she lived here so she can get the help I got. The staff is nice, courteous and always treated me wonderful and everyone showed genuine concern about my well-being which always made me feel very comfortable here."

Eugene A.

Age 79

Amityville, NY

Physical Therapy, Acupuncture and Epidural Shots Failed To Help By Low Back and Leg Pain...But the Relief Source Program Relieved the Pain and Made A Great Difference!

"Before starting treatment with Relief Source, I was very much in pain and limited in my activity. Everything I had already tried to help my back and leg pain FAILED including physical therapy, acupuncture and even epidural shots in my back. I chose to work with Relief Source because they offered something new and different from those other things. After completing the recommended program, which

included Warm Laser and Spinal Decompression therapy – it relieved the pain in my low back and leg to where now I'm able to do more activities with much greater ease and comfort. From where I was in the beginning prior to treatment to where I am right now, there is a GREAT DIFFERENCE and I would absolutely recommend this program!"

John B.
Age 81
Hicksville, NY

They Care About Their Patients And Only Want What's Best For Them!

I started treatment with Relief Source because I was suffering with pain and numbness in my left arm as well as neck pain. Their program made a lot more sense to me over getting shots or surgery. Now I can start my day knowing I'm doing better. I have more flexibility in my arm and neck and I have confidence again in myself! I would certainly recommend Relief Source to my friends and family. They are very professional and compassionate. They care about their patients and only want what's best for them. The office staff ladies are wonderful, also very professional and caring. Thank you!

Jim G.
Age 56
Lindenhurst, NY

Fixed My Radiating Arm Pain!
No More Numbness and Tingling In My Hands!

At 63, I have a history of cervical herniations. I was unsure of what I did to cause my cervical condition to worsen. I was in a lot of pain that radiated into my left arm with numbness and tingling into my fingers. The muscles in my arm were so sore that they hurt just from touching them. I could not keep my head up in the normal position. I was unable to drive a car. Lying down in the bed at night made the pain worse. Sleeping was impossible. I could not hold my head up enough to shave. Worst of all, I was not able to hold my grandson. Those harsh chiropractic adjustments weren't possible. I had to do something. I first saw and orthopedist who sent me for an MRI. He prescribed a painkiller which is addictive, but it reduced my pain only by about 10%, and even that small relief didn't last for very long. It wasn't worth risking addiction from this drug. He recommended that I begin epidural shots. I have had cervical injections a few years prior but found that they caused added pain instead of relief so more shots of any kind, to me was not an option. When the shots don't work, the next word that you hear is surgery. I was stuck between a rock and a hard place with nowhere to turn, or so I thought.

One day, my wife was on Facebook, and in passing by I glanced at the screen. There was a very prominent ad that I noticed for spinal decompression of the lumbar and cervical spine. I took this as a sign and called Relief Source. She kindly set up an appointment for me for a free consultation with the doctor. I had nothing to lose except for the pain and those addictive ineffective drugs and future painful injections, or possibly surgery. I had hope again that maybe this was the answer that I was looking for. My wife drove me in for the first consultation.

The doctor examined me and explained exactly was causing my pain and determined that I was a candidate for this type of treatment and proceeded to recommend cervical decompression combined it laser treatments for me. I left my MRI disc for him to review and we set up an appointment schedule for twice a week treatment. The decompression treatments are computer controlled and done at a very slow rate, which was a welcome relief to my already very traumatized condition. There was no pain at all during decompression as it is a very gentle treatment. The laser treatments are soothing, and the deep penetration also relieves pain. I had thankfully responded very quickly with this combined treatment and after only six visits, I was able to no drive myself to my remaining treatments. There is a lasting effect from each subsequent treatment that carried over the next treatment whereas you feel better and better as the treatments progress. Spinal decompression has a healing effect in the discs, rather than just masking symptoms as drugs and shots do. The combination of the electro stimulation with heat, and then gentle decompression and laser treatments has given me back a normal range of motion so that I can drive, shave, and most importantly hold my grandson again and all pain free. The doctor is very knowledgeable and easy going, friendly, efficient, honest, and thorough in his determinations of what your treatment options are and listens closely to your concerns and needs. He spends a lot of time with you. The office environment is very clean, peaceful, quiet and relaxing. The appointments are spaced and scheduled so that you almost never have to wait at all to be treated. I have recommended Relief Source to several friends, one which went for his free consultation and is already on the road to recovery with these pain-relieving treatments. This is my honest testimonial based on my own experience during my treatments. I have not been paid nor offered any special service or goods of any kind for my testimonial.

John K.

Age 63

Hewlett, NY

"I No Longer Have Shooting Nerve Pain Down My Leg And I'm Able To Stand WITHOUT ANY Type Of Pain!"

"Before I started treatment with Relief Source, I could not stand for more than 10 minutes without shooting pain down my left leg. I chose to have this procedure over other treatment options because I was seeing a pain management doctor and taking muscle relaxers and anti-inflammatories with no relief. Since I've had spinal decompression along with laser therapy I no longer have shooting nerve pain and I am able to stand without any type of pain. I would recommend this procedure to my friends and family. I had a very pleasant and relaxing experience at Relief Source. They showed concern about my well-being."

John L.
Age 69
Lindenhurst, NY

"I Was Suffering For More Than 5 YEARS...Now I am able to walk/stand the way I used to and the searing pain that used to plague me is GONE!"

When I started my treatment with Relief Source, I was at the end of my rope. I've been suffering with pain and stiffness for more than five years. Initially, all I did was get chiropractors treatment, such as T.E.N.S, stretching exercise, etc. Followed by acupuncture and massage therapy provided by a holistic medicine practitioner. All the aforementioned treatments provide short term relief and pain killers had no efficacy to this stubborn, ever-present pain which robbed me of the joy of living. I finally had a MRI on 2/14, which revealed that I had cervical issues such as posterior disk herniation and sciatica, but at this time no solution was offered to my problem, although I saw more than three orthopedic doctors. My only option was PT, I was told. In desperation I sought the help of a pain management doctor who injected me in three separate occasions, but the effect of that treatment was ephemeral. Finally, on February 2018, in desperation, acute pain and almost unable to walk I saw two or more doctors within one month! They both determined that I needed surgery ASAP. They even asked me "how are you able to walk?" Very slowly and painfully, I replied. In desperation I began looking for non-surgical alternative also due to utter fear of the surgery and the fact that I have yet to meet a person who's had surgery and it been cleared of PT, which I considered so prevalent and never-ending! That's how I came across this treatment during an online search.

The spinal decompression and the laser treatment made a remarkable difference from day one! The following visit I signed up for treatment without hesitation mostly due to the way the doctor explained his findings about my condition and how the treatment was going to address it. The treatment was god sent. I am able to walk/stand the way I used to and the searing pain that used to plague me is gone.

The contributing factors that made me elect the Relief Source treatment over surgery was that it was non-invasive, very pleasant and safe just as he mentioned. I love his office's atmosphere and his staff is very courteous, helpful and effortlessly friendly, truly formidable doctor's office. I will miss it now that my treatments finalized.

I will sincerely recommend this treatment and location to anyone I know who happens to be in need of the same treatment I received. I will be forever *indebted, they're very affable and concerned about patients progress as well as to the wonderful staff for being so caring and professional. God Bless.*

Carmen M.
Age 68
Bronx, NY

I Couldn't Perform Normal Activities or Even Work Due To The Low Back Pain...Now After Treatment My Back Is 80% Better and I'm A lot Happier with My Life Now!

"Before I started my treatment with Relief Source, on a scale from 1-100 my back was about 70% BAD. I couldn't perform normal activities or even work due to the pain. I first had tried acupuncture and then steroid injections which helped for a while, but in the end the pain just kept coming back. Now after my treatment, my back is over 80% BETTER. I can now do normal day to day activities like mowing and fixing my yard and I can even work now. I have more confidence and overall just feel a lot happier with my life now that I do not suffer from the pain I had before I started treatment. I would definitely recommend

anyone I know to see Relief Source to seek treatment for their pains. The environment in the office was great. The office was always clean, and everyone was very helpful and courteous towards me."

Tomas O.
Age 57
Bethpage, NY

Bibliography

1.   "What Is Sciatica: Sciatica Treatment & Causes. *Cleveland Clinic*." What Is Sciatica: Sciatica Treatment & Causes. Cleveland Clinic. N.p., n.d. Web.

2.   Ullrich, Peter F,, Jr., MD. "What's a Herniated Disc, Pinched Nerve, Bulging Disc…?" Spine-health. N.p., n.d. Web.

3.   "WebMD Arthritis and Joint Pain Center: Symptoms, Causes, Tests, and Treatments." *WebMD*. WebMD, n.d.

4.   "Bursitis Symptoms, Treatment (Shoulder, Hip, Elbow, and More)." WebMD. WebMD, n.d. Web.

5.   "Knee Bursitis Symptoms, Causes, Treatment - How Is Prepatellar Bursitis of the Knee

Treated? Are There Home Remedies for Knee Bursitis? – MedicineNet." MedicineNet. N.p., n.d. Web.

6. "Prepatellar Bursitis Symptoms." Arthritis-health. N.p., n.d. Web.

7. "Knee Tendonitis/Tendonosis." Sports Rehab and Chiropractic Care Washington DC Maryland and Virginia Knee TendonitisTendonosis Comments. N.p., n.d. Web.

8. "Patella Tendonosis | Sydney Sports Medicine Centre - Education." Patella Tendonosis | Sydney Sports Medicine Centre - Education. N.p., n.d. Web.

9. "Patellar Tendinitis." Symptoms. N.p., n.d. Web.

10. "Meniscus Tears-OrthoInfo - AAOS." Meniscus Tears-OrthoInfo - AAOS. N.p., n.d. Web.

11. "Torn Meniscus." Causes. Mayo Clinic. N.p., n.d. Web.

12. "Meniscus Tear Causes, Symptoms, and Treatments." WebMD. WebMD, n.d. Web.

13. "Meniscus Tear of the Knee." *Healthline.* N.p., n.d. Web

14. "Chondromalacia." *Healthline.* N.p., n.d. Web.

15. "Chondromalacia Patella (Patellofemoral Syndrome) Symptoms, Causes, Treatment - Chondromalacia Patella Facts - MedicineNet." *MedicineNet.* N.p., n.d. Web.

16. "Knee Sprain - How to Treat a Sprained Knee." Knee Sprain - *How to Treat a Sprained Knee.* N.p., n.d. Web.

17. "Knee Ligament Injuries. Knee Pain After Running | Patient." Patient. N.p., n.d

18. "Knee Osteoarthritis: Causes, Symptoms, Treatments." WebMD. *WebMD*, n.d. Web.

19. "Arthrosis Define, Causes, Symptoms Treatment, Difference." *Healthhypecom.* N.p., n.d. Web.

20. "Arthritis of the Knee-OrthoInfo - AAOS." *Arthritis of the Knee-OrthoInfo - AAOS.* N.p., n.d. Web.

21. "Iliotibial Band Friction Syndrome.": *Background, Anatomy, Pathophysiology*. N.p., n.d. Web.

22. "Nismat / Patients / Injury Evaluation & Treatment / Lower Body / Iliotibial Band Friction Syndrome Treatment." Nismat / Patients / Injury *Evaluation & Treatment / Lower Body / Iliotibial Band Friction Syndrome Treatment. N.p., n.d. Web.*

23. "Iliotibial Band Syndrome Symptoms, Causes, Treatment - Iliotibial Band (IT Band) Syndrome Facts - *MedicineNet." MedicineNet. N.p., n.d. Web.*

24. Mayo Clinic Staff. "Peripheral Neuropathy." Causes. Mayo Clinic, 04 Dec. 2014. Web. 22 July 2015. http://www.mayoclinic.org/diseases-conditions/peripheral-neuropathy/basics/causes/CON-20019948.

25. "The ReBuilder® Stops Pain While Treating Your Nerves - at Home." Safe, Effective

Neuropathy Treatment. Web. 25 July 2015. <http://www.rebuildermedical.com/>.

26. "Frequently Asked Questions." Frequently Asked Questions. Web. 25 July 2015. <http://www.rebuildermedical.com/frequently-asked-questions.php#chemo>.

27. Loghmani MT, Warden SJ. "Instrument-assisted cross-fiber massage accelerates knee ligament healing." Journal of Orthopaedic Sports Physical Therapy. 2009.

28. "Back Pain" Medline Plus. National Institutes of Health. 17 July 2013.

29. "Relief for Your Aching Back." *Back Pain*. Consumer Reports, Mar. 2013. Web.

30. David G. Borenstein, Sam W. Wiesel, Scott D. Boden. Low back and neck pain: comprehensive diagnosis and management, p. 41, 2004.

31. Dagenais S, Caro J, Haldeman S. A systematic review of low back pain cost of illness studies in the United States and internationally. *Spine*. 2007.

32. H. Paajanen, M. Erkintalo, R. Parkkola, J. Salminen and M. Kormano, "Age-dependent correlation of low-back pain and lumbar disc degeneration." *Archives of Orthopaedic and Trauma Surgery.* 1995.

33. Byron J. Richards, CCN. "Billions of Dollars Wasted on Medication Injuries." April 15, 2008.

34. LeBauer A, Brtalik R, Stowe K. "The effect of myofascial release (MFR) on an adult with idiopathic scoliosis." Journal of Bodywork and Movement Therapies. 2008.

35. J Bodyw Mov Ther. 2013 Oct;17(4):518-22. doi: 10.1016/j.jbmt.2013.03.001. Epub 2013 Apr 30. http://www.ncbi.nlm.nih.gov/pubmed/24139013.

36. MedlinePlus (June 7, 2012). U.S. National Library of Medicine. Medline Plus Trusted Health Information for You. Beta-carotene. Retrieved from www.nlm.nih.gov/medlineplus/druginfo/natural/999.html.

37. LL Magnetic Clay Inc.(1996-2010). Ancient Minerals:.Need More Magnesium? 10 Signs to Watch For. Retrieved from: www.ancient-minerals.com/magnesium-deficiency/need-more/.

38. WebMD.(2005–2012). Weight Loss & Diet Plans. Top 10 Iron-Rich Foods. Retrieved from: www.webmd.com/diet/features/top-10-iron-rich-foods.

39. More, J. (Sept. 2008). The British Dietetic Association. Vitamin D - The Unique Vitamin. Retrieved from: www.bda.uk.com/foodfacts/VitaminD.pdf.

40. Ferreira, Leonor Mateus. "Chiropractic Care May Help Control Peripheral Neuropathy in Diabetics." Diabetes News Journal. N.p., 16 Mar. 2015. Web. 27 July 2015. <http://diabetesnewsjournal.com/2015/03/17/chiropractic-care-may-help-control-peripheral-neuropathy-in-diabetics/>.

Made in the USA
Monee, IL
15 May 2021

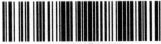